ALOE VERA

ALOE VERA

Nature's Legendary Healer

Alasdair Barcroft

Foreword by Hazel Courteney

SOUVENIR PRESS

First published 1996 by
Souvenir Press Ltd,
43 Great Russell Street, London WC1B 3PA

Reprinted 1997, 1998

ISBN 0 285 63352 X

Typeset by Rowland Phototypesetting Ltd,
Bury St Edmunds, Suffolk,
Printed in Great Britain by
The Guernsey Press Co., Ltd, Guernsey, Channel Islands.

Four vegetables are indispensable for the well being of man:
Wheat, the grape, the olive and aloe.
The first nourishes him, the second raises his spirit,
The third brings him harmony, and the fourth cures him.

Christopher Columbus (1451–1506)

You ask me what were the secret forces which sustained me during my long fasts. Well, it was my unshakeable faith in God, my simple and frugal lifestyle and the Aloe whose benefits I discovered upon my arrival in South Africa at the end of the nineteenth century.

Mahatma Gandhi (1869–1948)

During the 20 years that I have been treating my patients with Aloe, I have found that there are many diseases described by the doctors of antiquity which disappear rapidly when I administer Aloe in the form of granules or powder. Therefore, the good results which I have always obtained allow me to quote the adage of Roger Bacon:

'Do you wish to live as long as Noah?
Then take some pills of Aloah!'

François Vincent Raspail (1794–1878)

The doctor of the future will give no medicine but will interest his patients in the care of the human frame, in diet and in the cause and prevention of disease.

Thomas Edison (1847–1931)

Notice to Readers

All persistent symptoms, of whatever nature, may have under-
lying causes that need, and should not be treated without,
professional elucidation and evaluation. It is therefore very
important, if you intend to use this book for self-help, only to
do so in conjunction with duly prescribed conventional or
other therapy. In any event, read the advice carefully, and pay
particular attention to the precautions and warnings.

The Publisher makes no representation, express or implied,
with regard to the accuracy of the information contained in this
book, and legal responsibility or liability cannot be accepted by
the Author or the Publisher for any errors or omissions that
may be made or for any loss, damage, injury or problems
suffered or in any way arising from the use of aloe vera.

Contents

Foreword

Twenty years ago, whilst working as an air stewardess, I met a woman on a Caribbean beach who insisted I should buy some of her aloe vera for my sunburnt skin. To stop her continual pestering I agreed, and she deftly extracted the slimy gel fluid from the long cactus-like leaves and spread the sticky contents over my skin. She then proceeded to swallow what was left of the aloe liquid. I remember being completely horrified and asking if this was safe! She laughed and said that the aloe kept her young; she looked about 55 but said she was 72. I was very impressed and, much to my amazement, my red blisters healed within two days.

I never dreamt that one day I would become an alternative health writer who would write features about aloe vera, nor that I would begin drinking the juice every day of my life.

Alasdair Barcroft wrote to me at the *Daily Mail* in 1994 and told me that aloe vera was available as a stabilised drink and that he knew dozens of people who had used it to help heal various health problems. I was duly sceptical, as I receive hundreds of letters each week about new products and have learnt to remain impartial until I have seen and heard the evidence to back up the claims; however, my editor was sufficiently interested to commission a feature. During my research I interviewed nine top gastroenterologists and was astonished to find that only *one* had ever even heard of aloe vera.

Complementary medicine has come a long way even in the short time since I wrote that feature. Millions of people are literally sick of being sick, and fed up with the side-effects of taking long-term medication. Last year 10,000 people were hospitalised suffering side-effects from prescription drugs. We are at long last waking up to the power of prevention, the health insurance of the future.

Unfortunately, many of us take notice of our bodies only when they start to go wrong, and then often expect our doctors to give us a pill for our ills. The majority of us desperately need to take more responsibility for our health and to be more discerning about our diets. It's not our last meal that makes us sick, but our last thousand meals! Remember, our bodies are made up entirely of food molecules—if you put junk in, there is no doubt that in the long term the body will become ill. Junk foods have little or no nutritional value and the human body needs a regular intake of more than 50 essential nutrients to survive. Conversely, if you watch your diet and eat in a balanced way, you will reap the benefits.

Many family doctors are stressed and overworked; they are also bombarded with information from drug companies who are all too keen to increase their share in the lucrative prescription drug market. During five years at medical school most GPs receive no nutritional training and none in the use of supplement therapy. I have met hundreds of people who are now telling their doctors about alternatives, which include taking aloe vera juice to help conditions like psoriasis, eczema, arthritis, irritable bowel syndrome, constipation, exhaustion, ME and many other ailments. Some doctors remain sceptical, whilst others are taking note and are now openly suggesting dietary changes, nutritional supplements (vitamins and minerals) and other remedies, because they realise that many alternative treatments have enormous benefits, without the negative side-effects.

Whilst aloe vera cannot be termed a magic bullet for all our ills, it contains many nutrients that are vital to health. I take three tablespoons of high quality aloe vera every day in freshly made vegetable juice, and eat plenty of organic fruits, vegetables and grains. But I'm no saint—and often indulge in treats like home-made cakes and puddings! I also take quite a few supplements, as it is well proven that we cannot obtain all the essential nutrients we need from our diet for optimum health.

FOREWORD

Life in the '90s is full of potential hazards from pollution, pesticides, preservatives and additives like salt—not to mention the explosion in convenience foods, overuse of antibiotics, stress-related illnesses and allergic conditions. But nature and modern research are working hand in hand to offer us all the chance to stem the growing tide of disease and protect our bodies from today onwards. If you are reading this book, you are already on your journey towards renewed health. I wish you luck and light. Know that if you are willing to search, all the answers are out there waiting to be found.

Hazel Courteney
Journalist and author of
What's the Alternative?

Acknowledgements

I should like to thank all those people who have contributed to this book in their different ways, especially the following:

Hazel Courteney for kindly agreeing to write a foreword to the book and for her enthusiastic support over the past few years. Hazel is a successful journalist and author who writes a weekly column in the *Daily Mail* on alternative therapies. She has also published an A–Z of alternative remedies, *What's the Alternative?*, and I really believe that she has done more to put aloe vera on the map than any other journalist in the UK—indeed, when we first started talking to the press in 1994, she seemed to be the only one who was prepared to take us seriously.

Patrick Holford, founder of the Institute for Optimum Nutrition, for contributing to the chapter on nutrition and for permission to quote from his book, *Optimum Nutrition.*

Dr Greg Henderson, specialist in chiropractic, for his very helpful account of the ways in which aloe vera has benefited his patients.

Thank you also to Dustin Greene of Forever Living Products, who has been a great inspiration and source of help and advice, both to myself and to many people involved in the aloe vera industry in the UK. He has given me a new insight into the mind-boggling potential of aloe vera throughout the world.

Leo Spork of Pro-Ma Systems has shown an objectivity and total dedication to the cause of aloe vera which I have found very informative and refreshing. My thanks go to him, too.

An extra special thank you to Kate (Boss!) for her help and support at the most stressful time.

My biggest thank you is for my lovely and supportive wife,

Mary, and my great kids, Angus, Hamish and Helena, all of whom continue to be a source of joy and inspiration to me.

A. B.

Introduction

I first witnessed the healing powers of aloe vera more than fifteen years ago when, like Hazel Courteney, my younger sister was badly sunburnt in the Caribbean. A friend of hers treated her immediately with raw gel from a fresh plant and the relief and healing were, according to my sister, almost miraculous. This was one of those many lifetime incidents you simply store away in your memory and think no more of, although, as a family, over the years we regularly used products containing aloe vera.

Since establishing The Aloe Vera Centre, however, I have been amazed to discover the impact, that a so-called 'wacky cactus juice' can have on so many people's lives, and indeed on their quality of life. I had considerable difficulty in choosing the case histories for Chapter 6—there are just so many examples of people whose conditions have been helped by aloe vera.

This plant is not some magical panacea for all ills. It is a herbal juice which, when used fresh from the leaf or when properly stabilised and processed, seems to have powerful healing, anti-inflammatory, nutritional and general health-giving properties for both humans and animals. Although it should not be regarded as a cure-all, it does seem to help with a wide spectrum of apparently unconnected ailments and disorders. These range from arthritis, acne, asthma, athlete's foot, diabetes, cholesterol, hiatus hernia, sinusitis, eczema, ulcers and cold sores to IBS, ME, diverticulitis, ulcerative colitis, candida, constipation and conjunctivitis—and that's just the human story! For animals the list also seems endless!

Aloe vera was used for centuries by many civilisations to treat a host of internal and external ailments, long before the advent of modern medical practices and the development of

15

pharmaceutical drugs. Despite this, its 'magical' properties have largely been dismissed as folklore and myth by the 'conventional' medical fraternity, on the grounds that there is no 'significant clinical evidence' to support the hundreds of years of documented use and the growing wealth of current anecdotal evidence.

Since the 1980s, however, there has been a move (by both the medical profession and the general public) towards a more holistic approach to healing, with a greater emphasis on the use of natural products and alternative or complementary therapies. These treatments are steadily growing in popularity as the general public becomes more concerned about the long-term side-effects of some drugs and more aware of the role of improved nutrition, for example, in maintaining a healthier lifestyle. There is no doubt that this shift has become a trend and that aloe vera (provided it is of the highest quality) can play a significant role.

This book has been written as an accessible and factual introduction to aloe vera—what it is, what it contains, its properties, the type of products available and how they can be used, case histories of users and comments by therapists, what you should know before buying aloe vera and some handy hints and tips. It is certainly not my intention to promote any particular brand of aloe vera through the book and any references to brand names or specific products are generally confined to the chapters describing therapists' or individuals' own experiences with a particular product. Many of them may have tried different brands of aloe vera and found them to be either ineffective or less effective than those they have mentioned in this book.

People should become far more discerning about the quality of products they buy. Bear in mind the old saying, 'you pays your money and you takes your choice'. The use of the words 'aloe vera' on a product is no indication of its purity, quality or efficacy, nor does it offer any guide to the amount of aloe vera it contains. Potential buyers should take heed of the words of a well-known US grower of aloe vera who, when asked to comment on the proliferation of aloe vera drinks on the market (and this is now happening in the UK as well) said, 'If it looks like water, smells like water and tastes like water, it probably is water.' Having tried at least twelve different aloe vera drinks myself, I know there is a huge disparity in the pure aloe vera gel (essentially the active ingredient) content, the polysaccharide content and the purity and strength of the products currently on sale.

Nowadays some of the best brands of aloe vera tend to be sold direct rather than through shops, and customers should always do a little research before buying. Make sure you receive good advice on how to take the drink or how to use the topical products. Did you know you can now buy products with a ninety-day money-back guarantee? If such a guarantee is not forthcoming, you should look for an alternative.

I hope you enjoy reading this book and that it gives you a helpful introduction to aloe vera, a plant which I believe is only now really coming of age as we rediscover one of 'nature's legendary healers'.

CHAPTER 1

Ancient Myth or Modern Miracle?

No one can say for certain how long aloe vera has been known as a medicinal plant. One of the earliest recorded pharmaceutical uses of it can be found on a Sumerian clay tablet dating from 2100 BC but there are reports of drawings of the plant on Ancient Egyptian temple walls from as early as 4000 BC. It has been surrounded by myth and legend for so long that in some early cultures it acquired almost godlike status, being venerated for its healing properties.

Whatever the truth about its first recorded use, there is absolutely no doubt—it is well chronicled—that aloe vera played a significant and important role in the pharmacology of many early civilisations from the time of Christ onwards. There is considerable and undeniable evidence of the use of the plant as a wide-spectrum healing agent in places as far apart as Southern Europe, the Middle East, North Africa, Asia, the Far East and the Americas.

One of the most detailed early accounts appears in the Egyptian 'Papyrus Ebers', written around 1550 BC. This documented a number of formulae for the use of aloe (mixed with other natural products) in the treatment of various internal and external disorders.

The early Egyptians revered aloe and called it the 'Plant of

Immortality'. This may account for stories of its use in the embalming process (a procedure which apparently continues to baffle experts to this day) and for its importance in the burial rites of the Pharaohs, as well as for the tales of its use by the two Egyptian Queens, Nefertiti and Cleopatra. They were both renowned for their beauty and were said to bathe in its juices. Cleopatra's handmaiden is also said to have mixed it into skin lotions to enhance her mistress's loveliness.

The Israelites, after years of slavery in Egypt, may well have adopted some of their captors' funerary traditions, for legend has it that Solomon was an advocate of aloe and grew it for its aromatic and medicinal properties. The ancient peoples of Mesopotamia were said to have used the plant to ward off evil spirits from their homes, and, much later, the Knights Templar drank a concoction of palm wine, aloe pulp and hemp which they called the 'Elixir of Jerusalem' and to which they attributed their health and longevity.

By 600 BC aloe vera had reached Persia and India—probably introduced there by Arab traders. The Arabs by this time were using it both internally and externally and had discovered how to process the plant they called the 'Desert Lily' by using their bare feet to separate the gel and sap from the rind before emptying the resulting pulp into goatskin bags. These were set out in the sun until completely dried and the contents ground to a powder. Readers might be relieved to know that the processing of aloe vera these days has progressed enormously!

To this day the Bedouin tribes and the Tuareg warriors of the Sahara Desert know the plant as the 'Desert Lily'. From around 500 BC the island of Socotra (near the Horn of Africa) developed a reputation as a grower of aloe vera (one highly disputed legend claims that Alexander the Great conquered this island in order to ensure a continuous supply of plants to treat his wounded soldiers during his military campaigns). There are reputed to have been five plantations of aloe vera on Socotra and these were traded with countries as far away as Tibet, Malaysia, India and China.

The Hindus believed that aloe vera grew in the Garden of Eden and called it the 'Silent Healer'. Ancient Chinese doctors considered it to be one of the plants with major therapeutic properties and called it the 'Harmonic Remedy'. Incidentally, today the Americans also call it the 'Silent Healer' and the Russians, echoing the Ancient Egyptians, call it the 'Elixir of Longevity.'

In the Americas the plant was used for centuries by the Mayan people of Yucatan. The women used it to moisturise their skin and its bitter taste to wean their children off the breast. The Seminole Indians of Florida believed in its power of rejuvenation: the 'Fountain of Youth' for which Ponce de Leon, the explorer, searched in vain was said by them to spring from a pool in the middle of a cluster of aloe vera.

However, for the first real benchmark in our present-day understanding of the general use of aloe vera, we have to turn to the 'Greek Herbal' of Dioscorides (AD 41–68). This Greek physician developed both his skills and his knowledge while accompanying the conquering Roman armies of the time. He wrote what was probably the first detailed description of aloe vera as we know it today, noting that the contents of the leaf could be used for the treatment of boils and haemorrhoids, for healing the foreskin, to help soothe dry and itchy skin, for ulcerated genitals, for irritations to the tonsils, gums and throat, to help heal bruising and to stop the bleeding in wounds.

Another famous physician of that era, Pliny the Elder (AD 23–79), confirmed in his 'Plant History' the findings of Dioscorides but went further in establishing that aloe vera could help with numerous other ailments and could also reduce perspiration (could aloe vera have been the world's first antiperspirant?). Honey and rose oil were often mixed with it, maybe to counteract the bitterness and possibly because no one believed that the plant, on its own, could be such an effective healer!

During the Middle Ages and the Renaissance the use of medicinal aloe spread across the world and northwards into

21

Europe. Because it grew only in hot climates it was not under-
stood by the northern Europeans, although it grew widely in
Spain, Portugal and Italy where it was held in high regard.
Marco Polo is said to have written of the history of its passage
from the island of Socotra, along the trade routes to the countries of the Orient, and even Colombus, during his voyages of
discovery, noted its use on Cuba and on other Caribbean
islands, where it was used, amongst other things, for blisters,
insect bites and wounds.

Knowledge of the 'miracle plant' was passed down through
the generations by word of mouth, and where it grew indigenously it was revered for its medicinal properties and for its
seemingly magical powers of healing. Priests used it in many
religious rites and royal physicians wrote of its properties and
wide-ranging uses in their medical records. To the local people
it became a traditional remedy for numerous ailments, either
raw from the leaf itself or, if taken internally, processed by
boiling and/or drying.

In the fifteenth century aloe vera was 'discovered' by the
Jesuit priests of Spain. As highly educated scholars and physicians they had read the Greek and Roman medical texts
describing its properties and powers, and when they accompanied explorers to new countries they used the plant if they
found it growing there and planted it where none was available.
They carried their knowledge of aloe vera to various parts of
the Americas where they established missions following the
defeat of the indigenous Indians by successive conquistadors
and they are credited with spreading the cultivation and use
of the plant across much of what is now Latin America and
up into Mexico and Texas as they developed their mission
network.

There is little mention of aloe vera for the next two hundred
years except for medical references to *Aloe vulgaris* and 'bitter
aloes'. In the countries of northern Europe it was generally
used as a purgative when a violent but effective remedy was
called for, and this almost fearsome reputation, rather than

that of a healer, stuck for many years—even today some less well-informed people regard drinking aloe vera as hazardous, a conclusion based mainly on ignorance of the quality and purity of the products now available. The trade in the drug aloes, for use on both people and animals, continued until about the 1930s.

Its deserved reputation as a healing plant may actually have contributed to its failure in the more temperate parts of the globe—until recently. The reason was that as knowledge of aloe vera spread to these areas there was little or no understanding of the necessity to use fresh leaves in the balms and other healing products in order to ensure their purity, efficacy and, indeed, safety. It was therefore impossible to reproduce the seemingly 'magical' healing properties of aloe vera when fresh leaves were unavailable, and as a result, rather unfairly, it fell from grace. Over the years people became more and more convinced that the amazing healing powers of which they had heard so much were rooted more in folklore and myth than in reality.

So although in the hotter climates, where it grew in abundance, the plant continued to be used both for wounds and for a wide range of internal and external ailments, in northern Europe and North America it was pushed aside by the advances in modern medicine and the development of synthetic drugs. In the middle part of this century, however, there began to be a growing scientific understanding of the detrimental effect of oxidation on the quality and effectiveness of the leaf gel extract, and of the resulting vastly reduced medicinal and healing properties.

If aloe vera was to make a come-back, a technique had to be found to stabilise the gel and thus ensure that it could be used in a pure and safe form by people throughout the world. Various ways of processing were tried, but as they all included the use of the leaf rind and some used heat, they were either unwittingly compromising the healing properties or destroying most of the nutrients contained in the gel. Whichever technique was used, the substance, named in 1851 as 'aloin', which is the purgative agent found just underneath the hard green rind, remained.

It was not until the 1970s that scientists found an effective way of separating the aloin and the rind and then stabilising and thus preserving the gel taken from the leaf so that it was 'essentially identical to fresh gel'. A new chapter in aloe vera's history was about to open.

CHAPTER 2

Aloe Vera—
The True Aloe

There are more than 250 different known varieties of aloe, of which only three or four have significant healing or medicinal properties. The most potent of these, rich in vitamins, minerals, amino acids and enzymes, is *Aloe barbadensis Miller*, commonly known as aloe vera. The word 'aloe' is thought to be derived from the Arabic *alloeh*, meaning 'shining bitter substance', while 'vera' is the Latin word for 'true', because in ancient times this variety was regarded as the most effective for medicinal use. This book is concerned only with this variety.

Aloe vera, together with the rest of the aloe genus, grows only in hot climates and is found especially in the drier regions of the Americas, Asia, Europe, Africa and Australasia. It resembles a cactus in appearance but is actually a perennial succulent and a member of the Liliacae family, as are the onion, garlic, asparagus, lily and tulip. Aloe vera is characterised by long, hard, sword-shaped green leaves with sharp points and a seemingly fearsome array of barbs on each leaf edge. The leaves grow in a rosette pattern straight out of the ground and when the plant blooms in spring or autumn its bright yellow flowers appear high above the gel-bearing leaves, at the top of a leafless stem which grows out of the middle of the plant.

The genus aloe belongs to a larger class of plants known as xeroids, so called because they are able to close their stomata (minute openings in the epidermis of the leaf) to ensure that water is retained within the plant. This ability to conserve water allows members of the xeroid group to survive long periods of dry weather or even drought conditions. They also have the apparently miraculous ability (due to their special chemical make-up) to close any wound or damage to the outer skin almost instantly, thus preventing precious water from being lost. It is this power to heal itself that may have given ancient civilisations a clue to the potential use of aloe as a healing plant.

When cultivated for commercial use, the plant takes three to four years to mature, at which time the gel contained within the hard green outer leaf is at its most potent in relation to its nutritional content. When fully grown the outer leaves can reach a height of around 60–90 cms (2–3 feet) and weigh approximately 1.5–2 kilos (3–4 lbs) each. The larger leaves protect the younger leaves growing from the centre. The plants produce tiny replicas of themselves, called 'pups', which are carefully removed and planted in nursery beds. Every step of the cultivation and harvesting of the plant has to be done by hand to avoid damaging the leaves, for if the gel is exposed to the elements it will oxidise and thus lose its nutritional and medicinal benefits.

NATURE'S TREASURE CHEST

Aloe vera is a veritable storehouse of nutritional compounds— more than 75 have so far been identified by scientists. The list of vitamins, minerals, enzymes and amino acids reads like a 'what's what' of nutrition. Researchers are continuing to study the plant to try to unlock its secrets, but to date the conclusion seems to be that it is the synergistic way in which all the nutritional compounds work together that gives aloe vera its

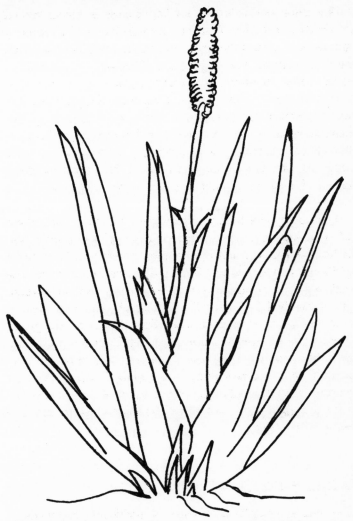

Aloe vera (*Aloe barbadensis Miller*) by Angus and Hamish Barcroft.

'magical' properties. No doubt, as technology develops further, the list of identifiable nutritional compounds and their associated benefits will continue to grow.

Enzymes—the Keys to Life

Enzymes are critical to human and animal life and their function is quite simply to break down the proteins in the food we eat into amino acids. These are then absorbed by the body and converted back by the enzymes into body protein. Enzymes essentially turn the food we eat into fuel for every cell in our body, so enabling those cells to function and our body to operate. However, what is it that fuels the enzymes and allows this ongoing complex chemical process to continue? The answer is vitamins and minerals, without which the whole process would come to a grinding halt. For example, the body cannot break down or utilise protein without zinc and vitamin B6. Vitamins B1, B2 and B3 (niacin) are essential for the production of energy.

Just as aloe vera's powerful healing qualities seem to be attributable to the complex and synergistic action of all its nutritional compounds, so the body is a complex of ongoing chemical processes and nutrient interactions. A good example of this is in the movement of muscles. In order for this to take place the body needs fuel—oxygen and carbohydrate—plus an array of vitamins and minerals, including B1, B2, B3, B5, calcium, magnesium and iron.

The vitamins A, C and E, plus the minerals zinc and selenium, are powerful antioxidant nutrients, whilst vitamins B3, B5 (pantothenic acid), B6 and B12, in combination with choline, calcium, magnesium, zinc, manganese, chromium, vitamins A, C and E and selenium, have a positive effect on brain function.

THE 'WHAT'S WHAT' IN ALOE VERA

Vitamins

A (beta carotene): for sight, skin, bones, anti-anaemia.
B1 (thiamin): for tissue growth and energy.

B2 (riboflavin): in combination with B6 produces blood cells.

B3 (niacinamide): helps regulate the metabolism.

B6 (pyridoxine): as vitamin B2.

B12 (cyanocobalamin): mostly found in meat and dairy foods, very rarely in plants, so is extremely beneficial for vegetarians/vegans. Lack of this can cause anaemia and certain neuropathological disorders.

C (ascorbic acid): fights infection by boosting the immune system.

E (tocopherol): with vitamin C it helps fights infection and aids healing.

(plus folic acid, vitamin B complex): the formation of blood.

Minerals

More than 20 minerals have been found in aloe vera, all of which are essential to health. They include:

Calcium and phosphorus: for teeth and bone growth.

Potassium (sorbate): regulates fluid components in the blood and muscles.

Iron: carries oxygen in red blood cells, helps body's resistance to infection.

Sodium: with potassium maintains balance of water and other body fluids and transports amino acids and glucose into body cells.

Choline: as a component of lecithin, needed in metabolism.

Magnesium and manganese: help maintain nervous system and muscles.

Copper: the formation of blood.

Chromium: facilitates blood sugar levels, glucose metabolism, circulatory system.

Zinc: boosts the immune system.

Mono- and Polysaccharides

The long-chain polysaccharides in aloe vera are believed to be vital components of its 'magical' properties. Monosaccharides are simple sugars which cannot be destroyed by water. See *Healing Properties*, p. 32.

Cellulose, glucose, mannose, aldonentose
Uronic acid, lipase, alinase
L-rhamnose
Acemannan: has recently been found to be helpful in the treatment of immune deficiency diseases such as cancer and AIDS.

A growing number of very experienced therapists, practitioners and doctors have worked with aloe vera for many years and seen its benefits in action. They believe that one of the major factors in the seemingly miraculous healing powers of the plant is its polysaccharide content. This means that the concentration of polysaccharides in a particular product could be directly related to its ability to provide healing and other benefits to the user (this would apply to both internal and topical products).

Essential Amino Acids

Amino acids are the building blocks of proteins and affect brain function, including emotions. They are important to every function of the body. 'Essential' means that the body does not manufacture its own.

Seven of the eight amino acids classified as 'essential' are in aloe vera, as well as a further eleven of the fourteen 'secondary' amino acids which the body creates out of another eight.

Isoleucine, leucine, lysine, methionine, phenylalanine: assimilation of proteins; pancreas and spleen, renovation of blood cells; prevent anaemia; help resistance to disease; liver;

digestion; muscle formation, insomnia; therapeutic use for depression.
Threonine, valine.

Secondary Amino Acids
Aspartic acid, glutamic acid, alanine, arginine, ½ Cystine.
Glycine, histidine, hydroxiproline, proline, serine, tyrosine.

Enzymes

Phosphatase, amylase.
Bradykinase: stimulates immune system, analgesic, anti-inflammatory.
Catalase: prevents accumulation of water in the body.
Cellulase: helps digestion of cellulose.
Creatine phosphokinase: muscular enzyme.
Lipase: aids digestion.
Nucleotidase.
Alkaline phosphatase.
Proteolytiase: hydrolyses proteins into their constituent elements.
Fatty acids: all unsaturated and essential for health. One, caprylic acid, is used in the treatment of fungal infections.

Lignin, Saponins, Anthraquinones

Lignin penetrates the skin easily but no one is quite sure what it does! Saponins are both cleansing and antiseptic. Anthraquinones have analgesic and laxative properties.

Aloin: antibiotic, cathartic.
Isobarbaloin: analgesic, antibiotic.
Anthranol.
Anthracene.
Aloetic acid: antibiotic.
Aloe emodin: bactericidal, laxative.

Cinnamic acid: germicidal, fungicidal.
Ester of cinnamic acid: analgesic, anaesthetic.
Etherol oil; tranquillising.
Chrisophanic acid: fungicidal for the skin.
Resistanol.

HEALING PROPERTIES

At a first reading the healing properties of aloe vera seem almost beyond belief. It is like being in a time warp, reading the list of wild claims for this efficacious plant being touted by some madly enthusiastic 'snake-oil' salesman at the end of the nineteenth century. Many people ask how a single plant can have such a wide range of benefits. How can aloe vera be one of the most efficient detoxifying agents, a powerful immune system stimulant, a strong anti-inflammatory agent, an analgesic, a stimulator of cell growth, an aid to the acceleration of tissue healing, an antiseptic, a rich source of nutrients and an aid to the digestive function—and be all of these simultaneously?

According to a leading US nutritionist, Dr Bruce Hedendal of the Hedendal Chiropractic and Nutrition Center, the key to aloe vera's power is that the plant is a rich source of a class of long-chain sugars known as mucopolysaccharides (MPS). In his opinion these are as vital to the body as bricks to a house. They are normally found in every cell in our bodies and we manufacture them ourselves in the first decade or so of our lives. Thereafter we rely on outside sources, and few plants are a richer source than aloe vera.

So what do these MPS's do? What function do they perform in the body? Could it be that they provide lubrication for our joints, that they line the colon, thus preventing the re-entry of toxic waste, and also, amongst other benefits, that they form a barrier against microbial invasion of the body's cells?

Acemannan

Aloe vera is especially rich in one mucopolysaccharide known as acemannan, which has recently been isolated by a US company, Carrington Laboratories. Acemannan works by interacting with the immune system, boosting it rather than overriding it. It is a potent stimulator of macrophages (white blood cells which destroy bacteria, tumour cells and so on) to produce immune agents such as interferon and interleukin. In 1990, at the third International Conference on Antiviral Research in Brussels, it was reported that acemannan had been found to inhibit the growth of implanted sarcoma in mice and that when tested on cats suffering from feline leukaemia, 80 per cent of the animals recovered—a complete reversal of the prevailing statistics.

As a result of this research, in 1991 the US Department of Agriculture (USDA) approved the use of acemannan in the treatment of fibrosarcoma in dogs and cats. Previously there had been no effective treatment for this cancer, but when exposed to acemannan the cancerous tissue is encapsulated and the tumour killed, thus facilitating surgical removal.

The unique mechanism of this key active ingredient, coupled with its direct antiviral activity, may explain why aloe vera shows such potential in treating a wide range of both human and animal ailments and diseases.

Believe it or not, the following benefits from aloe vera have all been testified to and witnessed by alternative therapists, medical practitioners and laymen throughout the world:

DETOXIFYING AGENT. When taken internally as a drink, aloe vera acts as a gentle cleanser and detoxifier (provided only the gel and not the aloin under the leaf rind is used), working throughout the digestive system and penetrating the skin tissue. It flushes out the dead skin cells, helps to regenerate new cell growth and promotes healthier tissue, thus accelerating the healing of wounds, lesions and ulcers. It will also have this effect when applied externally to broken skin.

DIGESTIVE FUNCTION. Dr Ivan Danhof, one of the world's leading authorities on aloe vera, believes that it can be generally beneficial to the entire gastro-intestinal system. A former professor of physiology at the University of Texas and President of North Texas Research Laboratories, he has acted as consultant to many of the world's leading pharmaceutical research institutes and has advised the US Food and Drug Administration. He maintains that due to its magnesium lactate content, aloe vera is able to lower activity in the stomach and is effective in reversing both occasional and chronic symptoms in the upper gastro-intestinal tract.

In his paper, 'Effect of Orally Consumed Aloe Vera Juice on Gastro-intestinal Function in Normal Human Beings', published in the US magazine *Prevention* in 1985, Dr Jeffrey Bland, of the Linus Pauling Institute of Science and Medicine in California, concluded from the results of a trial that aloe vera helps in the following ways: it improves the digestion without causing diarrhoea, it acts as a buffering agent to normalise the pH (like an alkalising agent), it reduces yeast content and promotes a more favourable balance of gastro-intestinal symbiotic bacteria. It can also help specifically with disorders such as indigestion, irritable bowel syndrome (IBS), colitis and acid stomach. He found that it could improve bowel regularity, and participants in the trial reported an increase in energy levels and an improved sense of well-being.

Other researchers have noted that aloe vera penetrates the wall of the digestive system, flushing out harmful bacteria and helping to repopulate the system with beneficial flora. Inflammation is thus reduced and there is an increase in the absorption of nutrients.

HEART CONDITIONS. Dr Danhof has found that calcium isocitrate salts in aloe vera can help people with heart problems or with a history of heart disease in the family. He recommends daily doses of the juice for those at risk. This finding has been endorsed by other researchers: in 1984, at the annual meeting of the American College of Angiology and the International College of Angiology, a paper presented by Dr O.P. Agarwal gave the results of a five-year study of 5,000 people diagnosed as having angina pectoris. After the 'husk of isabgol' and aloe vera were added to their diets they showed a marked reduction in serum cholesterol and the frequency of angina attacks was noticeably reduced. After five years all the patients were still alive and had reported no adverse side-effects.

Further studies have shown that daily doses of aloe vera juice can lower blood cholesterol by 12–14 points, and that blood pressure is lowered within a few weeks. What causes this latter effect is not yet known and research is currently in progress.

CANCER AND THE IMMUNE SYSTEM. As mentioned earlier, encouraging results have been obtained when treating cancer in animals with aloe vera, and it seems as if the plant can also benefit humans. Dr Danhof reports that aloe vera causes the release of tumour necrosis factor Alpha, which blocks the blood supply to cancerous growths, and a study at the Department of Epidemiology at the University of Okinawa in Japan found that daily doses of aloe vera could help prevent the onset of lung cancer in smokers.

In general aloe vera can have a remarkable effect on the immune system, stimulating, supporting and modulating. More specifically, it has proved beneficial to AIDS sufferers, helping to restore the T and B lymphocyte balance, and it is known to protect the immune function of the skin against ultraviolet radiation. A study at the M.D. Anderson Clinic at the Medical Center in Houston, Texas, considered the effects of ultraviolet exposure on the skin and found that when aloe vera gel was applied to the skin before testing, the immune cells were fully protected.

ANTI-INFLAMMATORY AGENT. Aloe vera is widely used in the treatment of such conditions as osteoarthritis, where it has a steroid-like action without the side-effects, and rheumatoid arthritis, and it can also reduce the redness, pain and swelling associated with muscular pain, sprains and strains, tendonitis and bruising. As I mentioned in the Introduction, I have myself seen its effectiveness against sunburn, and in her book *Herbal Medicine: The Natural Way to Get Well and Stay Well*, Dian Dincin Buchman suggests using it on burns, insect bites and stings, acne and poison ivy blisters. Indeed, rashes of all kinds will be soothed by an application of aloe vera gel to the inflamed area.

HEALING AGENT. We have already looked at aloe vera's ability to promote cell regeneration. This makes it a powerful healing agent for all types of wound, both internal and external. Dr Danhof notes that it can accelerate the healing of broken bones by stimulating the uptake of calcium and phosophorus—two minerals essential for healthy bone growth—and it is known to regenerate healthy skin tissue eight times more quickly than the norm. As a natural antiseptic, antibiotic and bactericide, it can clear up a wide range of infections, including those of fungal origin. Professor Patrick Pietroni, in *The Family Guide to Alternative Health Care*, advocates its use for athlete's foot, ringworm, thrush and vulvitis, and Ross Trattler, author of *Better Health Through Natural Healing*, recommends it for warts, verrucae and haemorrhoids, not to mention worm infestations. Dian Buchman has found applications of aloe vera effective in softening and breaking down patches of hard skin on the feet, hands or elbows.

MOISTURISER AND COHESIVE AGENT. Aloe vera is a uniquely effective moisturiser for the skin. It works in two ways: by its ability to carry nutrients and moisture down through all seven layers of the skin, so facilitating penetration and absorption, and, through its polysaccharides, by creating a barrier that prevents moisture loss from the skin. It is thus eminently suitable for people with dry skin, and because it contains an anti-histamine and an antibiotic it is also good for sensitive skins. These properties are all contributory factors in making it such a powerful healing agent.

ANTI-AGEING FACTOR. Dr Danhof has conducted studies to discover the secret of aloe vera's rejuvenating ability, and has found it in the plant's ability to increase production of human fibroblast cells between six and eight times faster than normal cell production.

Fibroblast cells are found in the dermis of the skin and are responsible for fabricating collagen, the skin's support protein which keeps it firm and supple. During sun exposure and through the normal ageing process, fibroblasts slow their collagen production, and as we grow older the quality of collagen is reduced and wrinkling becomes deeper. Dr Danhof found that aloe vera not only improved fibroblast cell structure but also accelerated the collagen-making process, and he believes the clue may lie, once again, with the polysaccharides and their moisture-binding properties. Many skin products which promise anti-ageing benefits do little more than temporarily hydrate the skin. They do not stimulate the production of natural collagen and the existing facial lines tend to remain as before.

Collagen production is not aloe vera's only contribution to the anti-ageing battle. As people grow older, many of them tend to develop ageing spots on the hands, due to a complicated chemical procedure in the body as well as to external factors like sunlight. Aloe vera, however, contains a potent blocker which can actually reverse this process by providing the skin with the components to rejuvenate itself at cellular level, producing younger, softer and more pliable skin. Dr Danhof tested the effect on his own hands by daily applications of aloe vera to one hand, leaving the other untreated. The difference was amazing: the untreated hand had numerous spots while the other was without blemish!

ADAPTOGENIC. This is the most extraordinary property of all, for aloe vera has the ability to act appropriately on the specific problem or problems of the individual using it. This is one reason why people respond to it in so many different and sometimes surprising ways. They might discover, while taking it for their asthma or arthritis, that their gums have stopped bleeding or that their skin has improved.

These are just some of the amazing properties of this apparently miraculous plant. One could also add that it helps to maintain the liver and kidneys in good condition and can even help to correct hepatic dysfunction, and that it has a beneficial effect on people with diabetes, working to reduce blood sugar levels and to restore the natural release mechanism. It is sad to have to report that so far all the research leading to these discoveries has been carried out in parts of the world other than the UK. This is perhaps because aloe vera—in the form required for testing—is very new in this country, and the majority of those working in orthodox medicine may either dismiss it out of hand or be very sceptical about the independence of any such research.

However, to end on a more optimistic note, aloe vera drinking gel has recently been the subject of clinical trials by one of the UK's leading equine vets for the treatment of post-viral syndrome in horses. The favourable results of these trials were published in the *Veterinary Times* of September 1996.

CHAPTER 3

Quality—The Essential Component

Walk into any health shop and you will find several brands of aloe vera juices, drinks and capsules arranged on the shelf. Most are in clear glass or plastic bottles and look like water. The labels suggest that the bottles contain between 95 per cent and 100 per cent pure aloe vera juice. The capsules claim to contain concentrated aloe vera, many times the strength of the juice. Phrases such as 'cold-pressed', 'whole-leaf aloe', 'double-concentrated' and even '50 times more concentrated than the standard' may be used. But what is the standard and what does it all mean?

Most of these descriptions are designed to make the consumer think that one particular brand is the best or the most cost-effective (the latter is a claim that people should consider carefully when thinking about their health). Some brands use labelling which is at best 'misleading', others use quotations, from acknowledged experts, which are out of context and were never meant to be used to promote that brand of aloe vera.

The acid test really lies in the quality of the aloe vera plants used and in the stringency of the manufacturing and processing standards, to ensure that 100 per cent stabilised aloe vera gel is the primary ingredient—this should be the most significant part, by volume, of any aloe vera product (I have tried products where the content of aloe vera, by volume, has varied from 10 per cent to over 96 per cent. I know which I would rather spend my money on). The stabilisation process must not involve chemicals and the purity of the product must be guaranteed from the time it is processed to the time it is consumed. Aloe vera products should also have a polysaccharide content of between 1,200 and 2,000 mg per litre—this is considered by Dr Danhof to be the spectrum within which one can expect optimum results.

Products may also have an accredited seal of approval, but most of them do not. The words 'aloe vera' seem to be appearing on soaps, shampoos, creams and lotions in every supermarket and chemist's, so how do you choose one brand rather than another and is the cost indicative of purity and quality?

WHY IS QUALITY SO IMPORTANT?

Aloe vera, like all living matter, decomposes. If it has not been treated properly soon after harvesting, it starts to lose its potency and therefore its efficacy. Unless it is handled carefully, some of the aloin may get into the gel and cause allergic reactions in some sensitive people and digestive problems in others. The leaf's inner gel should be the only part of the plant used. Aloin is contained in the red/yellow sap just below the rind. It has been found to have a strong purgative (laxative) effect and has a detrimental effect on cell growth.

The world's largest grower and processor of aloe vera owns thousands of acres of plantations where the plant is nurtured from the nursery beds right through to its use in the drinking gel and juices and in the creams and other products. The company observes the highest standard of production, and uses only the mature leaves from the *Aloe barbadensis Miller* plant, properly treated and preserved with a unique and patented stabilisation process.

Some companies subcontract the growing of the aloe vera plants to established independent growers who grow the plants to strict specifications using organic farming techniques. This ensures that no chemicals are ever used which could be detrimental to the purity of the finished product and its healing properties.

Smaller suppliers of aloe vera must buy their raw material or even finished product on the open market, with no guarantee that the leaf gel is still in the same fresh state as when it was harvested—in fact this is highly unlikely. It could well have lost some of its potency, either through oxidisation (decomposition) or from an inadequate process of preserving, using chemical rather than natural additives, or even from overheating the aloe vera during production, so destroying many of its nutrients (enzymes, amino acids, vitamins and minerals) and healing properties.

Aloe vera must be 'biologically alive' if it is to be effective, and using the right stabilisation process is critical. The largest growers and producers manufacture their products to the most exacting standards in so-called 'clean room' conditions to ensure that quality is consistent. Every batch is rigorously tested in accordance with strict and well established procedures.

GROWING ALOE VERA

Let's follow the plant from the nursery bed to full maturity.

Aloe vera should be grown organically, so no chemical sprays, fertilisers, pesticides or herbicides are used at any time throughout the cultivation process. At the moment there are thousands of acres of commercial plantations in Texas, Mexico, the Caribbean and Australia, as well as in the Far East to satisfy the burgeoning market in Japan, Taiwan, Indonesia, Malaysia and, of course, China, potentially the largest single market in the world. Because all the weeding and harvesting is done by hand these enormous operations are very labour-intensive.

In the nursery the 'pups', the small offshoots from the adult (rather like the common spider plants people keep in their houses), are planted by hand and nurtured until they are robust enough to be placed in the larger fields. They remain there for four years, being carefully tended until they reach maturity with their full complement of vitamins, minerals, amino acids, enzymes and the unique polysaccharides.

The leaves are then cut separately by hand, not machine, in order to avoid damaging the younger leaves in the middle of the plant. As the leaves grow and mature at differing rates and grow closely together, resembling a clump of celery, harvesting is an ongoing and careful process.

rind
(outer leaf)
red/yellow
sap with
aloin

```
————————————————————————————————————————
————————————————————————————————————————
XXXXXXXXXXXXXXXXXXXXXXXXXXXXXXXXXXXXXXXXX
XXXXXXXXXXXXXXXXXXXXXXXXXXXXXXXXXXXXXXXXX
-----------------------------------------
```

gel
and
pulp

```
————————————————————————————————————————
OOOOOOOOOOOOOOOOOOOOOOOOOOOOOOOOOOOOOOOO
OOOOOOOOOOOOOOOOOOOOOOOOOOOOOOOOOOOOOOOO
OOOOOOOOOOOOOOOOOOOOOOOOOOOOOOOOOOOOOOOO
OOOOOOOOOOOOOOOOOOOOOOOOOOOOOOOOOOOOOOOO
OOOOOOOOOOOOOOOOOOOOOOOOOOOOOOOOOOOOOOOO
OOOOOOOOOOOOOOOOOOOOOOOOOOOOOOOOOOOOOOOO
OOOOOOOOOOOOOOOOOOOOOOOOOOOOOOOOOOOOOOOO
OOOOOOOOOOOOOOOOOOOOOOOOOOOOOOOOOOOOOOOO
OOOOOOOOOOOOOOOOOOOOOOOOOOOOOOOOOOOOOOOO
OOOOOOOOOOOOOOOOOOOOOOOOOOOOOOOOOOOOOOOO
OOOOOOOOOOOOOOOOOOOOOOOOOOOOOOOOOOOOOOOO
OOOOOOOOOOOOOOOOOOOOOOOOOOOOOOOOOOOOOOOO
OOOOOOOOOOOOOOOOOOOOOOOOOOOOOOOOOOOOOOOO
OOOOOOOOOOOOOOOOOOOOOOOOOOOOOOOOOOOOOOOO
```

red/yellow
sap with
aloin (bitter
purgative

```
OOOOOOOOOOOOOOOOOOOOOOOOOOOOOOOOOOOOOOOO
————————————————————————————————————————
XXXXXXXXXXXXXXXXXXXXXXXXXXXXXXXXXXXXXXXXX
XXXXXXXXXXXXXXXXXXXXXXXXXXXXXXXXXXXXXXXXX
-----------------------------------------
```

rind
(outer leaf)

```
————————————————————————————————————————
```

This diagram shows the structure of the leaf and the close proximity of the sap containing the bitter aloin to the gel. It is important to ensure that the leaf rind and the layer containing the aloin are carefully separated from the gel, otherwise the bitter purgative could taint the purity and healing properties of the gel.

On arrival at the processing plant the leaves are transported on conveyor belts to an area where they are washed, topped and tailed, and then filleted. Much of this is also done by hand to avoid bruising or damaging the delicate structure of the leaf. The leaves are then cut lengthways and the clear gel removed. The rind is pulped down to be used as an organic soil conditioner and mulch for the growing crop, while the inner gel is collected and piped into vast stainless steel vats, each holding thousands of gallons. Here it goes through the process of stabilisation, a highly specialised technique using only natural ingredients.

STABILISATION AND PROCESSING

The producers of the highest quality aloe vera products manufacture them in accordance with the highest pharmaceutical standards, using stringent procedures to ensure that the aloe vera is not contaminated by aloin or any other substance, including the hard green outer rind. No chemicals are added and all products are made from food grade aloe vera and not from powdered concentrates.

The word 'stabilisation' is used by the largest manufacturer whose scientists developed a method of preserving the inner leaf gel. The process took years to perfect and is protected by two world patents. It guarantees that the 'stabilised aloe vera gel' and the raw gel from a mature leaf are 'essentially identical'. The complex technique is known not to interfere with the naturally synergistic working of all the gel's nutrients, and actually retains its freshness and enhances its healing properties so that they become more consistent.

Over the centuries households all over the world, even in colder climates, have had aloe vera plants growing indoors as a natural remedy to apply to cuts, burns and stings: by simply slicing the leaf lengthways to expose the gel and then rubbing it on the affected area, its cooling and healing effect can be felt almost instantaneously. Only in the last two decades, however, have products made from the gel become readily available to everyone around the world, wherever they live, from the North Pole to the South Pole and all points in between.

WHAT TO LOOK FOR WHEN BUYING ALOE VERA PRODUCTS

Track Record

I personally believe that this is one of the most important factors one should consider before buying anything. Most people would not dream of buying a car from a company with no track history! However, when it comes to something like aloe vera (and many other health products), because the unit cost is not that high they don't seem to care very much and in general spend far too little time, effort and money on their health compared to things like cigarettes, alcohol and petrol. If you want to be healthy you have to make an investment in that goal, so before you part with your money do some research.

There is a likelihood that aloe vera products purchased on a direct basis from companies which themselves control the growing of the plants and have track records stretching back nearly two decades will be far superior in quality to brands that are simply trying to take advantage of customer awareness and demand. The reason is obvious: they have stood the test of time, they have invested massively in research and development and have independent scientists monitoring all aspects of the growing and production cycles.

There are probably only two brands of aloe vera available in the United Kingdom from companies which control all aspects of the process, from the plants in the field to the retail customer. So far as I know those two companies are also the only ones that have a guarantee on their products. As I said in the Introduction, if in any doubt seek advice. I have seen so many people benefit from taking aloe vera, both internally and externally; just make sure, before you buy, that you have done your research and quality checks.

Polysaccharides

The world's leading authority on aloe vera, Dr Ivan Danhof (see Chapter 2), is quite forthright when he discusses the importance of these unique long-chain sugars and their benefits to both humans and animals. As stated earlier, the optimum polysaccharide content is between 1,200 and 2,000 mg per litre. The processing of the pure aloe vera should never compromise that concentration and no simple sugars or starches should be added to boost that level artificially. Concentration of the aloe vera can cause damage to the polysaccharides by both the processing and the increased concentration of natural salts remaining. Any change in the natural ratio of water to solids (99.5 per cent: 0.5 per cent) found in pure aloe vera gel or juice may have a detrimental effect on its range of benefits.

Patent

This is also important. A patent is only granted on a product or method (as in the stabilisation of aloe vera) which can be proved scientifically to be unique and to actually work.

Certification—Proof of Quality

The International Aloe Science Council (IASC)
This is an independent body which was set up to monitor standards and the quality of products within the aloe vera industry. Only those that meet its requirements are granted its Seal of Approval (see overleaf). This seal is on most brands of aloe vera products which are of the very highest quality and potency and means that they have been inspected and

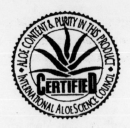

audited and that the products have been analysed. Independent experts use approved procedures developed by the IASC's Science and Technical Committee. At the time of writing the IASC confirms that the only brand sold in the UK which bears its Seal of Approval is Forever Living Products, a brand sold by direct retailing (as is that sold by Pro-Ma Systems) to the end user by trained independent distributors. The products are not available through retail shops. For further information about the IASC, see Appendix 1.

Kosher Rating
Another indication to look for on the container is the K mark (see illustration), a symbol of purity and quality that is known throughout the world. To gain this rating a rabbi from a certified laboratory inspects the processing facilities, the formula of the stabilisation method (in the case of aloe vera), the whole manufacturing process and the ingredients in the product. The standards set are rigidly high, and many religious groups, not merely those of the Jewish faith, see the Kosher rating as their guide to safer, purer products.

Islamic Seal of Approval
This also denotes a product of the highest quality and purity.

British Union Against Vivisection (BUAV)
The BUAV symbol or 'Bunny mark' (see diagram) tells you
that animals have not been used in the testing of these products.

**Not Tested
on Animals**

Is Price Indicative of Quality?

No, not at all. For example, a tube of aloe vera cream or jelly
costing a couple of pounds may contain very little aloe vera
and the quality may be debatable; even an expensive brand,
unless it was from one of the top manufacturers or had the
appropriate certification, might not contain any more aloe vera
or be of superior quality.

Can Some of the Labelling be Misleading?

In the UK, if a label says that the product contains a percentage
of aloe vera (let us say 95 per cent) you would expect the
contents of the bottle (or pot or tube) to be made up of 95 per
cent aloe vera, by volume.

In fact it may mean that there is as little as 10 per cent pure
aloe vera gel (or active ingredient) by volume but that the 10
per cent aloe vera content is actually 95 per cent pure. Confus-
ing, isn't it? In other words, I could claim that my glass of
water contains 95 per cent aloe vera, when in reality I have
added only a small amount of 95 per cent aloe vera to it. You
can perhaps understand why some people say they have tried
an aloe vera product and that they did not see or feel any
difference. So you cannot always rely on the label to tell the
whole story. However, what the label *may* tell you is whether
aloe vera is the principal ingredient in the product. It helps if

aloe vera is at the top of the list of ingredients—if it isn't, look for another brand.

Manufacturing processes, conditions and temperatures vary from company to company. In order to ensure that the biologically active ingredient is retained, temperatures must be strictly controlled and kept below certain levels and chemicals must not be added. For example, when buying a natural product like honey you should always make sure it is 'cold-pressed', which tells you that all the nutrients and other active ingredients are retained. The same is true of aloe vera—it is a 'biologically active' or 'living' food.

'Whole-leaf' aloe vera sounds like a desirable property but may not be—it depends how effectively the purgative (aloin) has been removed and whether, in that process, any of the beneficial nutrients have also been inadvertently extracted (see Appendix 1). As we have already seen, aloin, the bitter yellow substance found just under the leaf rind, is a strong purgative and in laboratory conditions it has been proven to kill cells.

The pure aloe vera gel, when properly stabilised and processed into a drink, has all the gentle properties needed to stimulate digestion in a safe, non-toxic and harmless way, but is also highly beneficial nutritionally and boosts the immune system.

What Does Aloe Vera Juice Look Like?

It is a slightly thick liquid (containing pulp) which is a dull creamy, yellowish colour. The colour can vary, naturally, from batch to batch, but some brands have been found to contain bleaches and artificial colourings to ensure that the colour is uniform in every bottle. And remember the US grower I quoted in the Introduction: if the juice looks like water and tastes like water there is a very good chance it will be mostly water. So again, look for another brand.

What Does It Taste Like?

It is an unusual taste, and I believe an acquired one. Some may find it slightly strange at first, though it does improve as your taste buds adjust. Good quality aloe vera is not necessarily sold for its taste!

Does the Design of the Bottle Give Any Clues?

It should be made from a light-deflecting substance, as otherwise the juice can deteriorate rapidly; clear glass or plastic will simply not do the job. The world's largest manufacturer uses specially developed plastic containers which have a triple membrane skin that prevents both oxygen and light penetrating the container. The drinking juice or gel inside has a shelf-life of up to five years, unopened (with the 'use by' date on the container); once opened it must be refrigerated and will remain usable for up to two months. Another leading manufacturer uses plastic containers which are impervious to both light and oxygen, and their products also have an extended shelf life.

To sum up, if you have any doubts about the quality, purity and effectiveness of any aloe vera product you are thinking of purchasing, do not buy it. If you write to or call The Aloe Vera Centre (see Appendix 1), they can provide advice on the best product or products for your particular needs.

CHAPTER 4

What the Therapists Say

Aloe vera is increasingly being recognised by alternative and complementary therapists as a natural way to cleanse and detoxify the body. When taken internally as a drink it is absorbed by the body, helping to promote healthier cells and hence healthier tissue. Given that our bodies replace around two and a half million cells per day, it is vital that those cells receive the maximum possible nutrition, and aloe vera can play an important role in that process.

Many therapists in the USA, including chiropractic physicians, have been using aloe vera, both orally and topically, for nearly twenty years; they believe it helps the body heal itself. In the UK, where aloe vera in a drinking form is comparatively new, it is making a significant impact on the way many therapists treat their patients.

This chapter records some of the comments, experiences and opinions of therapists in the USA and the UK, including examples of certain cases they have treated with aloe vera.

CHIROPRACTIC

Dr Greg Henderson, DC, FCTS, is a chiropractic physician and a multi-disciplinary nutritionist, and Director of Fallbrook Chiropractic Center in California. He has been using aloe vera as an integral and essential part of his patient care for over fifteen years. Here he details his views on aloe vera and its role in overall healing, good health and nutrition.

'Aloe vera is mainly known for its ability to inhibit pain. It is very easy to explain why it has this quality. It contains several analgesics and it can penetrate the layers of the skin, soothe the nerves and reduce inflammation.

'As an anti-inflammatory it has a property which we don't completely understand, causing it to penetrate the skin and fight inflammation. This is probably why many people seem to get positive results with inflammatory diseases such as arthritis. Aloe vera moves in and competes with the enzyme that causes inflammation, so that it does not spread or become any larger.

'Aloe vera also contains an ingredient that actually emulsifies cholesterol, thus enabling the body to eliminate it. It stimulates the cleansing and purifying of the blood in the liver and acts as a coagulator in cases of bleeding.

'Because it is a natural product which is recognised by the body and absorbed easily, people can achieve good results on comparatively small amounts. It also helps to speed the replacement of body tissue and makes the tissue better through healthier cell production. It contains uronic acids that actually strip away harmful materials from the body. Aloe vera also has an antibiotic effect which is well proven and well documented. Over the last twenty years we, in the western world, have developed and are routinely using superdrugs and, not surprisingly, have effectively created superbugs that are resistant. The interesting fact that I come across on a daily basis in my practice is that the high quality aloe vera I use is still effective against such organisms as salmonella, streptococci and staphylococci.

'One of the principal qualities of aloe vera is that it is a growth stimulator. For example, on a cut or burn it penetrates below the wound and promotes healing from the inside out. Because it replaces the fluids without stopping oxygen from getting to the wound, it helps to speed the healing processes and reduces the amount of scarring. Some of the hospitals in the US which are using aloe vera are having a 50 per cent faster rate of healing. In our practice we use it a lot with the cancer therapies, such as chemotherapy and radiation therapy, since it reduces the negative reaction of patients to the chemicals and the radiation. Our patients using aloe vera normally don't lose their hair, they don't get sick during those therapies and they respond much faster to the treatment.

'Aloe vera is a great energiser. If you drink it on a daily basis, you probably won't need as much sleep [this probably explains why the author can get by on between five and six hours' sleep a night and still has mountains of energy]. Not only is it a high quality nutritional product, but its healing power and value to the cells are among its greatest assets.

'In the intestines we can have many disorders, such as colitis and diverticulitis, and aloe vera has proved an excellent aid for all these: basically, it will work in any situation where there is an -itis (this means inflammation), so that is why it can help, because of its powerful anti-inflammatory properties, with such problems as arthritis, colitis, diverticulitis, etc. It has the ability to soothe, protect and cleanse the intestine, to detoxify the body and thus help to eliminate chemicals and other toxins which we get from the air and our processed foods.

'Aloe vera does not heal anybody! In all my years of practice and discussions with doctors I haven't met a doctor yet who has healed anyone! The body does its own healing—it just needs the right "vehicle". Aloe vera is known as the "healing plant" because it provides the body with the necessary things to take care of itself. For example, it can destroy the bacteria which cause peptic ulcers—up to 92 per cent of the time.

'One of the most remarkable examples that I have ever seen of the way in which it can accelerate the healing process relates to a plastic surgeon I know who uses what is effectively a chemical peel when performing face lifts. He uses a product called Aloe Activator to accelerate the recovery and healing time of his patients and has reduced this from six weeks to just over a week. This is a reduction by a factor of six and it shows just what can be achieved using the incredible healing powers of high quality aloe vera.'

AROMATHERAPY AND REFLEXOLOGY

Anoosh Liddell, MISPA, ITEC, is a reflexologist and aromatherapist who uses aloe vera to help in the treatment of a number of ailments, disorders and diseases. Here she outlines four of her more interesting cases.

Fatigue and Menopause

'Fay was 48 years old when I first saw her, and was in the early stages of menopause. She had unbearable sweats accompanied by hot flushes which were so bad that she had taken to going out into the garden at night in her nightgown and walking barefoot on the cold wet grass to cool off. Her GP had advised her to take hormone replacement therapy (HRT), which she did for a period of two months, but she was unhappy about taking HRT tablets as they raised her blood pressure and made her body bloat.

'She came to see me to find a natural way of alleviating her symptoms. I observed that she was overweight and had very dry body skin but oily face skin. Assessing her internal metabolism by reflexology methods, I found that she suffered from an incomplete emptying of the bowel and kidneys. Her general state of health was good but her body felt clogged, hence the fatigue and lethargy.

'I advised Fay to cut out drinking all tea and coffee and instead to drink two litres of pure still water per day and also four cups of dandelion herbal tea. This would start to flush out the kidneys and purify the blood and liver generally, and would also moisturise the body skin.

'Next I advised her to take aloe vera juice (50 millilitres

three times a day) and slippery elm powder (one teaspoon three times a day, mashed into half a banana) and also to take acidophilus and bifidus to enhance the friendly bacteria in her digestive system. This she had to do for three to ten days, eating nothing else except three portions of boiled rice (as little as possible). The object was for her to have three soft bowel movements per day before introducing a normal healthy diet very slowly over a period of three weeks or so. I tested her on her first visit with a full body massage and used clary sage, geranium, lemon and sage pure essential oils. I prescribed her a lotion of the same oils to apply to her lower back and abdomen each morning, and a blend of the same oils to use in the bath each night.

'One week later, when I saw her again, she said she had suffered all week with extreme headaches. This is a normal reaction of the body when it is going through a detoxification process.

'We continued working together and by the fourth week she felt wonderful. She has now been off HRT (her own choice and decision) for three weeks and has had only one mild hot flush. Her treatments are continuing and the progress she is making is extremely good. I have treated about six clients in this way and each one of them has shown wonderful results.'

Aids and HIV

'Working with people with AIDS is a very hard thing to do as we in complementary health care always struggle to help alleviate the awful side-effects of the powerful drugs which have to be used to keep opportunistic infection at bay. The main body systems which are affected by these drugs are the digestive system (which includes the whole alimentary canal, from the mouth to the stomach, liver, pancreas, intestines and bowel) and the urinary system (kidneys and bladder).

'Aloe vera juice taken each day (60 millilitres three times a day or more) soothes and repairs the damage done to these internal organs, giving the person less constipation, stomach cramps and burning urination, and promoting healthier skin. Although by no means a cure, aloe vera, combined with total holistic aromatherapy, has proved to be extremely helpful in improving the quality of life for many of those suffering with HIV and AIDS.'

Psoriasis

'The first case of psoriasis I treated was in a young child aged seven. Her psoriasis was mainly confined to severe scalp infliction and also bad itchy scabbing behind the ears. Her mother had visited the doctor regularly for three months asking for help, as the child was scratching her scalp so often, causing bleeding, and she was scared of infection. The usual shampoos and steroid creams were applied but there was little or no relief.

'I recommended a gentle change in the child's diet—slowly eliminating all dairy produce, convenience foods, white flour products, all fizzy drinks and pickled foods and all oranges and tomatoes. As psoriasis is related to the nutritional integrity of the skin and the health of the skin as a whole is dependent on the nutrients that reach it from the blood vessels in the body's connective tissue, aloe vera juice was the main ingredient I used to relieve the psoriasis.

'The nutritional value of aloe vera would in this case correct any increased body needs for certain nutrients which were not being supplied and possibly creating a deficiency, so resulting in psoriasis symptoms. I also prepared an oil blend containing jojoba, sweet almond, evening primrose, sesame seed and borage oils, together with essential oils of benzoin, bergamot, cajuput, neroli, birch and rose otto, to be massaged into the scalp and behind the ears each night, and then washed out with a mild vegetable-based shampoo the following morning.

'As a tonic after washing, I prescribed a few drops of a blend of essential oils (bergamot, carrot seed, german chamomile, eucalyptus and lavender) mixed in 100 millilitres of water in a plant sprayer, to be applied to the damp hair, making sure the scalp was well moistened. The child's hair was left to dry naturally. This treatment of oiling, hair tonic and aloe vera was continued for one week.

'Within two days all the scabs had lifted and come away, leaving behind soft new pink skin and no itching whatsoever. As the weeks passed the child continued to take aloe vera each day, but the need for the hair oiling and spraying grew less until it was done only once a week. A year has now passed and the child is still totally free of psoriasis.'

Eczema

'I had been regularly treating older children and adults who had minor attacks of eczema from time to time, but had never seen such bad eczema as in a four-year-old child I treated recently. Almost her entire body was covered, and her arms and legs needed constant covering up to stop her scratching them, causing bleeding and the added risk of infection. Her mother was very concerned, as each time she went back to her doctor another stronger dose of cortisone cream was prescribed.

'I suggested that she bathe the child each day in spring water to which Dead Sea salt had been added, and thereafter should apply pure aloe vera juice with a soft pastry brush all over her daughter's limbs and anywhere else where the eczema was apparent. Small sips of aloe vera juice were given throughout the day and wild blue-green algae as well.

'At first the eczema got worse, but I recommended that she persevere as I felt sure the condition would improve. It took six months before changes were noticed, and during this period I also recommended a slow but quite drastic change in diet as the food intake of the child was particularly high in cow dairy products, sweet, sugary foods and drinks and white flour products.

'Both mother and child suffered much during this adjustment period, but the results were well worth all the effort. Once the eczema had settled down and was only very mild, I made up a liquid blend of aloe vera juice and essential oils of geranium, german chamomile, juniper, sandalwood, lavender and myrrh to be applied all over each night after a bath. The eczema has not totally gone, but there has been at least a 90 per cent improvement, allowing the child to go happily to nursery school.'

NUTRITION

Venetia Armitage, DTH, is a registered nutritionist who has been taking aloe vera and giving it to her patients, mostly as a general health drink tonic, for about five years. Recently she discovered a new brand and realised the significant difference in the quality and gel content and the impact that could have on her patients by giving it to them in a more concentrated form. She describes here how she uses it.

'For their initial consultation I usually suggest that my patients take aloe vera along with a cleansing, high-vitality diet. The aloe vera soothes and heals the gut, encouraging good bacteria and rehydrating the system.

'Although the body will always try to heal itself, without good tissue and sufficient fluid it is difficult to achieve any significant results. With its ability to hold onto water, aloe vera is able to keep the body moisturised so that healing can begin. Once the body is cleansed and rehydrated it can better utilise vitamins and minerals from food and supplements.

'As the majority of my patients have digestive problems, and some are very debilitated, aloe vera is invaluable for relieving pain and discomfort and easing the painful spasms caused by problems like irritable bowel syndrome (IBS). Many IBS sufferers swear by their daily dose of aloe vera, in some cases eventually being able to dispense with their medical drugs. I use aloe vera with the utmost confidence, having seen it change the lives of many of my patients who have benefited so much.'

MEDICAL HERBALISM

Rosemary Titterington, M.I.Hort., is the founder and owner of Iden Croft Herbs in Kent, an internationally renowned centre for aromatic and medicinal herbs. She comments on the benefits she has found from using various products containing aloe vera.

'For many years I myself have used, and recommended to others, the natural juice of the aloe vera plant. It has proved invaluable when used in the home, as a leaf can be removed and the juice used for first aid on burns, blisters, skin irritations and insect bites. However, it is not the most convenient plant to take in your luggage when travelling! I was thus delighted with the convenience of pure ''aloe vera juice in a tub''.

'From my own experience and from verbal reports from our customers I have found that Aloe Vera Gelly is good for burns, providing good, quick first aid on clean, cooled skin (I apply cold water first to reduce the heat), and for treating blisters from burns. My daughter burned her foot on a hot water bottle, and a dressing of aloe vera beneath a 'ring pad', for protection, prevented the huge blister from bursting, reduced the swelling and the wound healed without a scar.

'I have used or recommended it for eczema, dry skin (particularly for older ladies), sunburn, insect bites, heat rash, nettle rash, and so on. It appears to be soothing and reduces itching.

'Some customers have found Aloe Vera Jojoba Shampoo very useful for dry, itchy scalp conditions, psoriasis and so on, and generally useful with sensitive skin and dry hair. Aloe Lip Salve is also very good for dry lips caused by wind and weather.

'I recommended to a group of people with Parkinson's disease that they try drinking the juice and the feedback has been very promising. I know that some of the Parkinsonians are still using it, and some of the carers have also found it beneficial for them—it helps to reduce the problems caused by tension.'

STRESS COUNSELLING

Kate Ker, MBAFATT (Member of the British Association for Autogenic Training and Therapy), is a stress counsellor who uses and recommends aloe vera.

Cystitis and Acne

'One of my clients was having a bad attack of cystitis. She was under a lot of stress and was drinking lots of coffee to keep her going. After a week of drinking Aloe Vera Gel twice a day her symptoms had gone. She also applied Aloe Vera Gelly topically whenever she visited the bathroom, which she said gave immediate relief locally. However, she noticed that the tube wasn't going to last very long and remarked on it to her sixteen-year-old daughter, who admitted that she was using it on her acne which covered her face, upper chest, upper back and shoulders. More tubes were acquired and they too were used quickly. It transpired that her brother was using it for his acne, too! The good news was that within a matter of only six weeks they didn't have a spot between them!'

IBS

'I first became aware of aloe vera from a client whose main problem was irritable bowel syndrome. This is a very painful complaint: the bowel goes into spasm and causes severe constipation interspersed with bouts of severe diarrhoea. The symptoms would flare up particularly badly when she was under stress or if she had eaten very refined foods like pre-cooked meals, white bread or white rice. The Aloe Vera Gel, taken as a drinking juice, was immediately soothing and would bring her bowel movements under control within about 24 hours. The symptoms did not recur if she stayed on the aloe vera every day, but would return if she came off it for a few days.'

NUTRITION, HOMOEOPATHY AND AROMATHERAPY

Adrian Blake has been involved in complementary medicine for many years. He describes here two of his most recent cases involving aloe vera and its benefits.

'Jenny is a 48-year-old housewife who came to us for homoeo-pathic counselling. For twelve years she had been going to see her GP, complaining of pains in her stomach, but although numerous tests were done, nothing could be found. She was admitted to hospital for further investigation.

'On opening up the abdomen and examining the internal organs there appeared to be haemorrhaging from various sites but no cause could be found, so as a routine the appendix was removed.

'Unfortunately, two months later the pains in her stomach recurred and she went back to her GP who again referred her to the hospital. This time it was decided to remove her spleen. For the next eighteen months she made various trips to her GP and back into theatre for exploratory operations, and she also had her gall bladder removed. Each time the haemor-rhaging improved temporarily and then returned six to eight weeks later. It was therefore as a last resort that she came to us for help.

'We looked at Jenny's case history and decided that there had been so much shock and trauma that she needed a remedy to restore the balance. She did seem to be quite poorly nour-ished, had trouble absorbing and digesting many foods and her appetite was poor. It was decided to try some aloe vera juice as a way of healing the internal organs in her body as much as possible with the micronutrients that are in aloe vera.

The juice would also increase the life force and energy of her organs internally.

'Initially we started her off with as much aloe vera as she could tolerate without causing a loose bowel. Some days she would consume up to half a litre of stabilised aloe vera gel, taking small amounts throughout the day. After a few days she reported that her bowel movements were much more regular and over the next couple of weeks her appetite improved. Within a month she seemed to be a much brighter, stronger, more centred person altogether.

'She continued with the treatment for the next three months, during which time neither the pains nor the haemorrhaging recurred. We can only assume that she was able to absorb the nutrients and take the healing from the aloe vera and therefore restore her body to normal. She is now capable of absorbing and digesting nutrients from everyday foods and is naturally very pleased not to have to return to her GP or to hospital for further exploratory operations.'

'The second case concerns Gerry, a fitness fanatic aged 38, who used to weight-train several times a week. Unfortunately his problem appeared to be the result of over-exercise! He had exercised his abdomen so much that it seemed to have gone into spasm. This had left him bedridden for a couple of weeks and unable to do any exercise. Unfortunately, while this was happening—while his abdomen was in spasm—the colon became underactive. So normal viruses, parasites and bacteria that would routinely be eliminated by daily bowel movements began to build up and he experienced extreme pain and discomfort every time he tried to have a bowel movement. This situation continued and it soon became extremely ulcerated. He also discovered that he could not pass anything that was at all abrasive without experiencing pain.

'After about a week bleeding ensued and the combination of this, the ulceration and spasms continued for several more weeks. He then went to his GP who gave him some painkillers, told him to rest and indicated it would heal up in a few days. The problem continued for the next month and there was no evidence of any healing. Gerry came to us in desperation for homoeopathic counselling. As soon as we saw his condition we knew something needed to be done quickly to alleviate the widespread inflammation and pain in the abdominal area.

'We put him on aloe vera gel drinking juice immediately to reduce both the inflammation and the pain and to help heal the ulceration and thus stop the haemorrhaging. He initially started on a few tablespoons and found that it was very soothing, allowing him to have a bowel movement more freely and without as much pain. Within two weeks the haemorrhaging stopped. He tried increasing the dosage slightly over the next few weeks and found that he was again able to tolerate the foods that had previously given him so many problems.

'Gerry had also become slightly anaemic and lethargic because of his experiences. However, over the next few months he found that, apart from healing his abdominal problems, the aloe vera was acting like a tonic on the rest of his system. Aloe vera is what we call a ''universal healer'' and acts at a cellular level to help heal and regenerate healthy tissue. He was able to resume his gym activities within a few months, stronger and fitter than he had been before the problem began. This is a fine example of the complete breadth and depth of what a high-quality aloe vera juice can do.'

SPORTS-RELATED INJURIES AND PROBLEMS

Although in the USA aloe vera products have been used extensively for nearly two decades, to help with a wide range of sports-related injuries, there has yet to be the same widespread acceptance of the plant's benefits among UK sports therapists. With the impact of increased professionalism and massive cash investments in more and more sports, therapists in the UK will be under increasing pressure to find new ways to accelerate the healing process and get injured athletes and players back into action.

Edward L. Clarry, MFPhys, specialises in sports injury treatment and exercise physiology. By chance he read an advertisement for aloe vera juice, which recommended its use in sports medicine. He began to use it in his clinic, with some remarkable results. Here he describes two cases he has treated successfully using aloe vera products.

'Robert is a 27-year-old American Footballer. He had a massive contact haematoma (bleeding within the muscle) of the left thigh which extended to the ankle, an infected Astro Turf burn over the left knee, inflammation and grazing to the right shin. He came into the clinic supported on two crutches and could not straighten or bend his leg. The injury was one week old and X-rays had confirmed that there was no fracture. The hospital had advised rest. Normally I would expect this type of injury to take between six and ten weeks to heal. I used ultrasound with aloe vera gel pulsed at 1.5m for five minutes, and Aloe Compression Wrap with intermittent compression for 25 minutes, and advised him to take aloe vera juice (30 millilitres four times per day). I also prescribed some remedial exercise.

'After the first treatment he was able to straighten his leg and walk without crutches. Three days after the second treatment the bruising was clear over the treated area and the burn infection was healing. He played American Football in the third week. After just four weeks and the fifth treatment, the injury was completely healed, as was the Astro Turf burn.

'I was particularly pleased with this result. Direct impact injuries of this kind can be complicated. If immediate treatment is inadequate, deep located intramuscular bleeding may gradually become calcified, which can lead to myositis ossification, a lengthy inflammatory process which normally requires treatment over a long period of time or surgical removal of the ossification.

'The Aloe Soothing Aid Spray healed the Astro Turf burn in a fraction of the time normally expected. With this type of burn, due to secondary infection, it is quite common for the injury to last all season. I have never seen a single case of secondary infection when Aloe Soothing Aid Spray has been used in first aid treatment, and the burns normally heal in a few days. When the injury has been infected due to lack of adequate first aid care it has healed in one or two weeks after treatment with the spray.

'The second case was Helen, a secretary aged 37 who had not worked for two years due to injury. She had fallen from a step-ladder and had fractured her foot and ankle. She had undergone surgery, during which a steel plate and steel pins had been inserted, followed by physiotherapy at the hospital.

'After two years Helen could not move her foot, ankle or toes and was suffering from extreme pain when walking. The foot and ankle were swollen, discoloured and inflamed. She had not worn normal shoes for two years and needed a stick for support. Her foot was very sensitive to the touch, indicating nerve irritation or pressure.

'I applied Aloe Compression Wrap with intermittent compression (25 minutes each treatment), Aloe Massage Lotion and Aloe Sports Spray after the foot became less painful to the touch. I also recommended her to drink 30 millilitres of aloe vera juice three times a day as an anti-inflammatory, and to apply Aloe Vera Compression Wraps when she went to bed at night. It was important that she should try to exercise the foot and ankle as her condition improved, so I gave her a progressive routine to follow.

'There was an improvement in the swelling and soreness after the very first treatment, with a progressive improvement after each subsequent treatment. In just three weeks and after six treatments, the pain, tenderness and swelling had reduced considerably, with the shape of the ankle reappearing. The dark brown discolouration had changed to pink and I was able to apply pressure in massage.

'Limited movement returned in her foot, toes and ankle. The limitation was due to calcification—not surprising after two years' lack of treatment. At four weeks she was walking without sticks and has now bought new shoes after two years. She informed me that the orthopaedic consultant had stated that he had not expected her to regain so much movement and advised her to keep on with the treatment.

'My patients are now recommending aloe vera to their families and friends. They are claiming some incredible improvements in well-being, performance, energy, niggling ailments clearing up, improvements in arthritic conditions and skin problems. They also report some 'unbelievable' improvements in conditions such as IBS, colitis and ME. I have found that Aloe Massage Lotion, when massaged into the cervical, thoracic and lumbar spine regions, can be very useful in relieving the symptoms of back pain, especially when the Sports Spray is also used as part of the massage programme or as part of ultrasound or interferential treatment, and also as a part of a self-treatment programme. Aloe Wraps are very effective for knee and ankle injuries as part of a compression programme. Aloe Ice Block Massage after applying heat packs gives good results as part of a hot and cold treatment.

'Aloe vera products are now a very essential part of my changing room and field first aid kit.'

Athletes and players of many different sports in the UK, as well as a few therapists, are now beginning to realise the incredible healing powers of aloe vera. For those who have any doubts, I would recommend they read a book called *Healing Winners* by Bill C. Coats and Michael 'Spanky' Stephens, in which the authors discuss ways of using a number of aloe vera products to help treat a range of different problems.

CHAPTER 5

Nutrition—You Are What You Absorb

Here in the Western world we are the best fed but the worst nourished. We have found ways to strip our food of valuable nutrients while simultaneously ensuring that it stays in our bodies for longer than is necessary, clogging up the digestive system and either fermenting or decomposing there. Not a comforting thought!

We need plenty of roughage in our diet. For centuries a close eye has been kept on our bowel movements. In days of old the reigning monarch would have had his or her very own (very personal) servant, and doctors who would examine the royal stool daily in order to gauge the health of their royal patient. Nowadays, many doctors and nutritionists believe that sickness and disease are caused by a sluggish, overworked and ineffectual bowel.

Take a bowl of brown rice. Naturally, each grain has a husk which is rough-coated, and this is where most of the nutrients are stored. When eaten and chewed well the nutrients are extracted by the time the rice has been broken down in order to pass through the colon. There, the colon's muscles move in gentle waves (peristalsis) pushing the rice (as was) along to the bowel. The husk provides the bulk and roughage which trigger the peristaltic movement, so cleaning the sides of the colon and the bowel and ensuring complete elimination, which means that everywhere is left clean and tidy with no bits left behind to cause bacteria to form.

Now take a bowl of white rice. While being processed the husk is taken away, which is what is meant by 'polished' grains of rice. All that are left are a few nutrients (most of which will be lost in the cooking) and a lot of sticky starch. The roughage has gone along with much of the food value. This spoonful of refinement is eaten, sits for not very long in the stomach doing nothing much (the worst thing for someone trying to lose weight) and ends up in the colon, a sticky mush which cannot trigger the peristaltic waves in quite the same way because there is not enough fibrous bulk.

It meanders slowly along to the bowel, leaving sluggish bits and pieces clinging stickily to the tiny crevices in the walls. These pieces decompose, causing bacteria to form and the body's defence to leap into attack, fighting off the threat of infection. By the time the rice has been eliminated it has possibly caused some problems along the way. The debris it leaves behind can cause diverticulitis, irritable bowel syndrome, bowel cancer and, of course, leads to poor absorption of nutrients.

Obviously, if someone is living on a diet consisting only of highly refined and processed foods like white rice, white flour and precooked meals from the supermarket, and is not eating sufficient roughage from vegetables and fruit, the above scenario is repeated daily, perhaps over many years, and the body simply gets exhausted from trying to extract a small quantity of nutrients while struggling to eliminate the waste.

The even worse news is that all the chemicals from pesticides and fertilisers used on cereals, vegetables and fruit gradually have an effect on our immune systems anyway—but that's another story!

It's no wonder that with this constant daily bombardment of chemically refined food our systems become tired and depleted, and it shows in our skins. Eat too much chocolate and stodge, add too much stress, which demands a quick boost of extra nutritional energy for the body, and skin soon becomes greasy or dry, puffy, blotchy, spotty ... I could go on!

The food we put into our bodies has the vitamins, minerals, proteins, carbohydrates, and everything usable extracted from it so that the body can turn them into energy to fuel every system inside our skin. Put aloe vera into our bodies and we have an unpolluted, organically grown, fibrous pulp, rich in valuable nutrients. Because of its deeply penetrating action on the skin, working first on the digestive system, then from system to system, it gradually helps the body to flush out the impurities and toxins and to restore balance to both overworked and sluggish areas. In time the inner health starts to show on the outside.

On average in the UK, trainee doctors spend less than thirty hours studying the subject of nutrition, and this is over a five- to seven-year learning period. This is quite astounding in itself, and when one also considers that there is a growing realisation amongst healthcare professionals and nutritional therapists alike that a significant percentage of cancers and many other killer diseases can be linked to diet, one has to ask the questions, what is being done to improve the situation and what can I do to improve my own situation?

This chapter is not designed to be a guide to nutrition—there are many eminently qualified people who write papers and books on the subject every day—but to highlight the fact that people need to start thinking more seriously about what they eat and drink and whether their daily diet regime should be altered. They also need to know that any nutrients and supplements they take are of the right quality and in an absorbable form.

I believe aloe vera can play a part in improving a person's overall nutrition and well-being, but it is not some 'nutritional panacea' that one can switch on and off like a light switch to make up for the lack of a healthy diet and lifestyle.

Recently, when I read one of Patrick Holford's books, *Opti-*

mum Nutrition, I really began to understand the words of Dr Carl Pfeiffer (who is referred to in the book) when he said, and I quote, 'It is my firmly held belief that with an adequate intake of micronutrients—essential substances we need to nourish us—most chronic diseases would not exist. Good nutritional therapy is the medicine of the future. We have already waited too long for it.' This from a brilliant scientist who, at the age of 51, had a massive heart attack and was given a maximum of ten years to live, provided he had a pacemaker fitted. He chose not to and then spent the next thirty years of his life researching and developing optimum nutrition.

Let's put it to the expert.

I asked Patrick Holford, the pioneer of optimum nutrition in the UK and the founder of the Institute for Optimum Nutrition in London, to contribute to this chapter because he is best qualified to discuss the importance of nutrition and the role aloe vera can play in establishing and maintaining a healthy nutritional lifestyle. I am convinced that if more people listened to what he says and acted upon it, they would not only lead a healthier and more active lifestyle, they would be better nourished and more able to cope with the rigours of present-day life. Here are his comments.

Every single cell in your body is made from the food you eat. For this obvious reason nutrition is considered the cornerstone of health. This is also why Hippocrates said, more than 2,000 years ago, 'Let food be your medicine and medicine your food.'

As the science of nutrition advances, we discover more and more naturally-occurring substances in food that are necessary for good health. First there were carbohydrates, protein and fat; then vitamins and minerals; then enzymes; then essential fats; then antioxidants and now 'phytochemicals', a catch-all phrase for chemicals found in plants which have positive effects on our health and resistance to disease.

Nutraceuticals or Pharmaceuticals?

Parallelling the increasing realisation that what you eat has the greatest effect on your health is the increasing realisation that the causes of most of the diseases we suffer from stem from the fact that we are moving increasingly further away from our natural design. Currently, the conservative estimate is that *seventy-five* per cent of the diseases we die from are diet-related. Many of today's diseases are being shown to be the accumulated result of toxic agrochemicals, drugs, food chemicals and eating a highly processed diet. Yet in most cases, the treatment recommended involves a cocktail of pharmaceutical drugs, substances completely alien to the human body, with undesirable side-effects. At the thin end of the wedge, modern-day living and eating are causing fatigue, decreased resistance to disease and stress and a whole lot of other 'minor' health problems that make life less than satisfactory.

Recently I rang up two doctors who had been in general practice for many years. One told me, 'I'm convinced that nutrition will be a major part of medicine in the foreseeable future. I'm getting substantially better results with diet and supplements than I used to with drugs.' The other said, 'The evidence for nutritional therapy is becoming so strong that if the doctors of today don't become nutritionists, the nutritionists will become the doctors of tomorrow.'

Instead of using pharmaceutical drugs with undesirable side-effects, the medicine of tomorrow is turning to nutraceuticals, nature's pharmacy of nutrients found in living foods, to correct the body's chemistry and restore well-being. A plant such as aloe vera contains such a cocktail of proven health-promoting substances that to isolate each ingredient and then treat it like a drug to cure a specific illness is not only impractical, it is nonsensical.

Aloe vera contains over one hundred vitamins, minerals, enzymes, antioxidants and important phytochemicals. Recently, the effect of one antioxidant, vitamin E, was shown (by a large-scale medical study carried out by Cambridge University) to be three times more powerful at reducing the risk of a heart attack than the best available drug. Just think what the effects would be of a lifetime of eating living foods, fruits, vegetables and nature's most action-packed health promoters like aloe vera. Plants like this provide a whole cocktail of essential vitamins, minerals, amino acids, antioxidants, enzymes and phytochemicals that work together synergistically to promote good health. Not surprisingly, the proven beneficial effects of aloe vera are very diverse, making it an excellent all-round tonic.

Research by Dr Jeffrey Bland has shown that aloe vera juice improves digestion, the absorption of nutrients and elimination. As well as all the nutrients within the juice there is a special factor that is attracting a lot of attention. This is a complex type of carbohydrate called a mucopolysaccharide, or MPS for short. As we saw in Chapter 2, MPS's are a major building block for the human body. They also help to boost the immune system. In animal studies, the MPS's in aloe vera have been shown to be powerful anti-cancer agents, stimulating the production of macrophages, which fight off cancer cells.

A lack of MPS's means the gut wall becomes too 'leaky', letting through large food molecules which we can then react to allergically. So anyone with an 'irritable bowel' or inflammatory bowel condition like colitis can benefit from aloe vera. The increased leakiness of tissue means an increased risk of infection and allergy, so people who are allergic or get frequent infections can be helped. MPS's are also natural anti-inflammatory agents, so they tend to calm down inflammatory diseases like arthritis, asthma or eczema.

You Are What You Can Digest and Absorb

Many raw foods contain the enzymes needed to break the food down, but these enzymes are often destroyed by cooking. Aloe vera is especially rich in digestive enzymes, so unlike cooked

71

food which taxes the body, aloe vera assists the body to break foods down. Since it also helps to promote a healthy digestive tract, it improves absorption of nutrients. Aloe vera is, itself, rich in nutrients including the vital antioxidant nutrients, vitamins A, C, E, selenium and zinc, to name a few, which are proven to protect us from heart disease and cancer, to boost the immune system and slow down the ageing process. Aloe vera also contains two per cent essential fatty acids which are needed by the brain and nervous system, the skin and almost every organ of the body. Once again, cooked foods contain mainly damaged or 'hydrogenated' fats, while processed foods use these or saturated fat. These hard fats are the ones that can kill, while the essential fats have the power to heal.

I believe tomorrow's medicine will be about using nutrients instead of drugs. It will be about looking through a new pair of glasses which reveal the true causes of disease. In most cases these lie in faulty nutrition, pollution, stress, and lack of exercise—the greatest cause of all being *ignorance*.

As Thomas Edison, the great inventor, said, 'The doctor of the future will give no medicine but will interest his patients in the care of the human frame, diet, and the cause and prevention of disease.' As modern science is now proving, *nature already has the answers. Living food like aloe vera, uncontaminated by man-made chemicals, contains all the ingredients we need for promoting health and vitality.*

CHAPTER 6

The People Have Their Say

This chapter describes the personal experiences of many people who have found that aloe vera has played a role in helping to alleviate the pain or other symptoms of the ailment or condition from which they suffer. We are certainly not suggesting that anyone with any sort of medical problem should stop taking prescribed medication. We are simply reporting the observations and comments of those who have found aloe vera helpful. In some instances, using aloe vera has significantly improved their quality of life after many years of suffering. It is not a cure, but it can help the body to heal itself. The accounts have been selected from the hundreds of letters received by the Aloe Vera Centre, Forever Living Products and Pro-Ma Systems. Names and locations have been changed to protect the privacy of the senders.

*   *   *

John had been an IBS sufferer for nine years when he was introduced to a new brand of aloe vera drinking liquid. Within weeks he felt better, and to give some idea of the beneficial effect, he explains here what living with IBS had been like.

His symptoms are typical of those experienced by many IBS sufferers.

'The causes and effects of IBS vary from individual to individual. I personally react badly to alcohol, spicy food, rich sauces and citrus fruits, made all the worse if I feel under stress. The effect of these on me is severe distension of the gut, causing a lot of internal pressure and, in some situations, extreme pain. From this I would suffer either bad constipation or diarrhoea, each causing as much discomfort as the other. I tried various so-called remedies, including prescriptions from the doctor for a drug to help with bowel spasms, peppermint oil capsules and a bulking gel, none of which ever seemed to have any positive effect.

'I spent more money going to a homoeopathic doctor, whose prescribed diet definitely seemed to help; however, after nearly two months of being unable to touch alcohol, spicy foods and other enjoyable food and drink, I couldn't stand it any more! I really believe that because of the very nature of IBS, if the medication or treatment regime is inconvenient or restricts your eating or other pleasures, it is unlikely that you will stay with it for long.

'What I have experienced with this aloe vera juice is that, despite the fact that it doesn't taste too great, it is very convenient and, most importantly, I can now enjoy the food and drink that used to upset me so badly.

'I take about two full tablespoons morning and night (i.e. four tablespoons per day) and I have experienced a huge difference in the way I feel. I have been taking aloe vera for nearly two years and in that time I have felt better and fitter than at any time in the last twelve years. I can quite confidently say that aloe vera has enabled me to enjoy a more or less pain-free life.'

Jane, who lives in Cambridge, read about the benefits of aloe vera for IBS in her newspaper and found that it cleared up the problem in three months. But she found that aloe vera helped her in other ways, too:

'Being over seventy years old I had a few complaints, and asthma was one which I contracted in 1986 and which is treated with steroids. To my surprise, I realised I was using my inhaler less frequently: the Aloe Vera Gel drinking juice was also keeping the inflammation down, helping me through chest infections.

'The ultimate happening was a hip replacement in 1996, combined with sensitive skin resulting from steroid treatment. My legs became very dry, scaly and sore, and once again I turned to aloe vera products—in this case Aloe Liquid Soap and Aloe Moisturising Lotion which I found invaluable.'

Michael is in his late forties and is a director of a UK-based multinational engineering company. As a child he had severe asthma and bronchitis, and he was not expected to survive past the age of eleven. He did and it was subsequently discovered that he was allergic to a wide variety of things, especially grass pollen. He had various treatments over the years, including anti-allergy injections which left him with a lung which is approximately ninety per cent efficient compared to normal. As he grew older the impact lessened, but in winter particularly he has had to use a combination of inhalers, one to dilate the lungs and the other to control local infection.

Within a few months of first taking Aloe Vera Gel drink he realised that he was no longer having to use either of the inhalers, and this has now been the case for more than nine months. In the last fifteen years he has never had such a long usage gap. Previously, he was also prone to fairly frequent sore throats in the winter which he believes were related to his respiratory problem, and these too have now disappeared. He still travels abroad frequently and is in a high-pressure and fairly stressful job—all things that can bring on an asthma attack. Although he still carries the inhalers he now never has need to use them.

Michael's case is by no means unusual. Many people with asthma report similar effects and say that by drinking Aloe

Vera Gel or Juice, or Aloe Berry Nectar, they have been able to dispense with their inhalers. It does not happen overnight, however, so anyone considering using aloe vera should ensure that it is of the highest quality and should persist with it for several months to see if it can help.

In 1994 Diana was suffering a very stressful period in her life and at the same time developed very severe stomach cramps and headaches. Thinking the worst, she consulted her GP who suspected IBS but suggested that she visit a consultant who in turn ran a series of tests on her stomach. There appeared to be no medical reason for the extreme discomfort and he therefore diagnosed IBS and prescribed a course of tablets. Diana explains what happened next:

'By a stroke of luck, the following day I read an article in the newspaper on the benefits of aloe vera, featuring someone who was a very severe sufferer from IBS. As the address given was very near to my own office, I made an appointment and went directly by taxi and obtained the Aloe Vera Gel that same day. Within a few days of taking aloe vera I felt better and have never looked back, although very occasionally certain foods may trigger an attack. Not only has it helped my IBS, but my general health and well-being have greatly improved.

'I have recommended aloe vera to many of my friends and relations, not only for IBS but for various other reasons, and they all confirm they would not do without it now. Surprisingly enough, my husband has had symptoms similar to IBS for the last couple of months and is at present going through various tests for elimination. I started him on aloe vera immediately and he is greatly improved, but of course, to be on the safe side he is continuing with his tests. I have also used Aloe Vera Gelly and Aloe Vera Heat Lotion which in turn were great for stings, sunburn and muscular pains.'

Rosemary has had chronic IBS for ten years and during that time has suffered from severe constipation, diarrhoea, stomach cramps, bloating and general discomfort. When she had her first two children, before she was introduced to Aloe Vera Gel, these symptoms became worse. Anybody who has been pregnant will know that trying to go to the lavatory can be very uncomfortable, but, as Rosemary explains, with IBS it's even worse:

'I used to get spasms quite unexpectedly, and if this happens when you are out you have to find a loo very quickly. I used to get panic attacks at the prospect of not being able to find a toilet, so it tends to restrict what you do and where you go. About a year before my third child was born, I read an article in a national newspaper that suggested aloe vera could help with digestive disorders. I haven't looked back since. I have taken Aloe Vera Gel every day and my third pregnancy was so much easier. All the bloating and spasms disappeared within a couple of months of starting the aloe vera and I was able to go to the loo without any discomfort. Talk about a major breakthrough, the relief was just brilliant!

'All through my third pregnancy and since being on aloe vera I seem to have had much more energy and consequently haven't felt as tired as I did in my previous two pregnancies. Also, if I ever get a tummy bug (and this is much less frequently than I used to) when I am abroad on holiday, I seem to recover much more quickly now than I did before.

'I have three young children and also run a charity granting wishes for terminally ill children, which can be very demanding, both physically and mentally. Taking aloe vera has changed my life for the better—I am so much improved that even my husband, who has watched the transformation, has now started to take this plant 'elixir'. I have recommended it to all my friends as a tonic and if they do have any sort of digestive disorder I have suggested they try aloe vera. For all you pregnant ladies out there I recommend you try it, but just make sure it's pure '100 per cent stabilised Aloe Vera Gel drinking juice.'

*   *   *

When Simon was a child he suffered quite badly from asthma. After a while it improved, but in his thirties it came back again, which he found extremely frustrating. Then he was introduced to aloe vera and was told to take about three table-spoonfuls of a drink called Aloe Berry Nectar every morning as a general tonic and energy booster.

'After a couple weeks I realised that I was wheezing less, as well as having increased energy, so I rang my niece to find out whether aloe vera could possibly help asthma. "Yes," she said, "didn't I tell you?" Six months later I really stopped taking my inhaler altogether. The interesting thing about it was that I didn't even know aloe vera could help asthma, so it wasn't a question of mind over matter.

'Having been off the inhaler for over a year, and free of asthma, I recently went on a two-week sailing holiday without my aloe vera. Within a few days I had a recurrence of my asthma and had to purchase an inhaler locally. However, on returning to the UK and restarting my aloe vera juice the asthma disappeared again and hasn't returned, and I no longer need to use my inhaler. What an amazing natural drink.'

For nine years Natalie had been waging a war with candida albicans. This left her with constant thrush, fatigue, acne, tissue and joint inflammation, as well as food, chemical and pollen allergies and intolerances. Then a year ago she started taking aloe vera and has noticed a steady improvement in her health:

'I now drink Aloe Vera Gel twice daily, which soothes my irritable bowel and bladder, eases my fatigue and improves my energy levels considerably. Aloe Vera Gelly is excellent for acne, painful joints and gingivitis. The Aloe Propolis cream and hand cream (Aloe Moisturising Lotion) are excellent for eczema, as well as for sunburn.

'I believe, however, that Aloe Activator is the most versatile of all the products I have tried. As a mouthwash, it soothes sore and inflamed areas, reduces inflammation and inhibits bacterial and fungal growth. For sinusitis and hay fever, it can be trickled into each nostril and sniffed. It makes your eyes water but works well. For sore throats, again it can be trickled into the nostrils and allowed to run down the back of the throat, or it can be gargled. It stings initially but stops the soreness in its tracks. For earache, trickling some into the affected ear works wonders. It has even made a slight difference to my mother's hearing loss!

'Either activator or gelly can also be used on a tampon to ease vaginal discomfort from thrush and I imagine would also help dryness if that was a problem.

'All in all I have found aloe vera products an all-round and very necessary and successful aid to my body's journey in regaining its good health and I shall be forever grateful.'

While Sheila and her husband were living in Cyprus, from 1987 to 1990, their son, then aged four, developed a skin problem on his face—extremely dry flaky skin on both cheek-bones, just below his eyes. To begin with they tried various mild moisturising creams but the problem became worse, spreading to the sides of his ears and up into his scalp. When they returned to the UK on home leave, Sheila took him to a GP who looked at the problem and prescribed a steroid cream for his face and another liquid for his scalp. The cream, when applied, turned the dry white flaky skin into bright red, shiny, sore-looking skin, making the problem seem even worse. Sheila continues the story:

'We persisted with the cream, hoping that in time it would begin to take effect. The liquid was so strong that it was hurting his head, so we stopped using that altogether. The cream didn't help at all, so we took him back to the doctor who then prescribed another treatment—this time a very mild aqueous skin cream, which didn't work either. This was the first of many visits and umpteen different treatments, over a period of five years, during which time the skin problem continued to worsen. We tried all sorts of creams and numerous different products were prescribed; none seemed to have any positive effect.

79

'During this time he was being continually teased at school because of the dry scaly skin on his face and the dry skin on his scalp, which looked like very bad dandruff. Prior to this problem he had always liked a very short crew-cut hairstyle, but with his scalp looking as though it was covered in dandruff he wanted his hair kept longer to hide the problem.

'The children at school began calling him "dandruff face" and saying that he didn't wash his hair enough. As you can imagine, he was hurt by their taunts and was well and truly fed up with the whole business.

'In 1994 we were introduced by my sister-in-law to a new range of products, made from aloe vera. We decided to try the Aloe Propolis cream on his face since, being pure and chemical-free, it certainly couldn't do any harm, unlike some of the prescribed treatments which contained steroids. We put the cream on his face three times a day, when possible, and were astonished at the outcome.

'Within four to five days there was no trace of dry skin anywhere on his face. We couldn't believe that the problem had cleared up so quickly, especially after five years of to-ing and fro-ing to various doctors, trying all sorts of different creams in an attempt to sort it out.

'Before trying the Aloe Propolis cream we had been referred to a skin specialist, so we decided to use the cream on his face only, leaving his scalp as it was for the specialist to see and hopefully diagnose the cause of the problem. We were so impressed by the success of the Aloe Propolis cream that we took a tube with us, to show the skin specialist what we had used to cure the facial problem. The specialist looked at my son's scalp and suggested he might have nits, much to my indignation as I knew for a fact that this wasn't the case.

'She took skin samples and said she would contact us the following morning. When she phoned—no nits in evidence (we could have told her that!) but she didn't know what the problem was—another scalp treatment was prescribed, a shampoo which we decided not to bother with as we had no intention of starting the same rigmarole all over again.

'We decided to use more of the products from my sister-in-law, namely the Aloe Jojoba shampoo and also the Aloe Rinse conditioner on his scalp, rather than the shampoo prescribed to us by the specialist. After only a few shampoos we saw an incredible improvement and decided to continue using the two products. His scalp condition is now totally healed and has remained so for two years, as has the problem on his face. My son rarely gets a chance to use the products now as all the rest of the family use them!'

Just before turning 30 Jessica moved to London after several years in Inverness where she had worked as a psychotherapist, teaching a stress management technique called autogenic training. When she was offered a job with a leading London stress expert she jumped at the chance, believing that she could adapt to life off the Euston Road after the wide open spaces of Glen Affric, the crisp clean air and the warmth of her friends and neighbours. However, as she describes, she was proved wrong:

'I became obsessed with work, then realised I needed more exercise. I took up T'ai Chi, rode several times a week, swam regularly, played bad tennis, wore my terrier's paws down to the bone and tried jogging, too. Oh, and I also became a vegetarian without any basic knowledge of nutrition.

'I moved to Sussex in order to benefit from the fume-filled journey to and from London every day! By the time I got home at 9.30pm I'd be too tired to cook, so I would open yet another can of beans.

'When I was 33 I had a series of tummy bugs—sickness, diarrhoea and loss of appetite. The last bout was the worst, leaving me too weak to stand.

'I struggled on, noticing that I became exhausted by lunchtime, couldn't practise my T'ai Chi for longer than a minute or so at a time, and, far worse, I discovered one day that I couldn't 'rise to the trot' or concentrate on simple instructions given by my riding teacher; an easy figure of eight became an insoluble problem of geometry. I was also a danger to shipping at the local swimming baths. This went on for a year.

'ME was eventually diagnosed by a homoeopathic practitioner, after my GP had given up more traditional tests. Homoeopathy got me over that initial crisis but I was increasingly frustrated and anxious about my future. My savings were being used up on treatments and I just couldn't work the hours I used to. Over the next eight years I tried many different approaches to the problem. I learnt to work within 70 per cent of my energy limits, not to over-exert myself physically (without much success as it's very difficult to know in advance when there's no prior warning), and to eat often to keep blood sugar levels balanced. I was also told to relax more—in other words I had to take a dose of my own medicine, a chastening experience.

'Two of my clients had told me of the benefits of a health drink called Aloe Vera Gel. They told me it was full of enzymes, essential amino acids, minerals and vitamins—many of the B ones, including B12. It works internally to detoxify the system and has been known as a healing plant for thousands of years. Just what I needed, I thought. That was nearly a year ago.

'The Aloe Vera Gel drink took some getting used to; it's certainly not sold for its taste and for the first few weeks some of my old ME symptoms flared up again, but they passed and I gradually started to improve. My skin colour returned after years of being waxy white, and I found that some stamina was there to back up the increased energy. I still eat regularly, but if I am out and miss a meal it's rare that I have a severe energy drop. My digestion is smoother and quicker and my hair has come back to life. Oh, and I've lost over a stone and a half without trying!'

Judy is forty-two years old and started suffering from ulcerative colitis in her thirties. At first she was given steroid enemas and Sulphasalazine tablets. She was allergic to the Sulphasalaz-ine, so was put on Asacol which she has taken ever since. After a while the steroid enemas could no longer cope as the condition worsened, so she was put on steroid tablets. The amount she took varied, 10mg a day being about average, but she had great difficulty getting below 5mg a day without having a flare-up and then having to increase the dose. Here Judy takes up the story:

'My consultant spoke to me several times about surgery which seemed the only way out, but he agreed I could have a while to try alternative remedies. I had already tried aroma-therapy and reflexology and various homoeopathic remedies but none of these had done much good. I was very depressed, constantly tired and I had also developed a fistula in my colon. I suffered from chronic pain, diarrhoea, bleeding, always rush-ing to the loo (and scared of not being able to get there in time). I was also terribly fatigued and was very nervous of going out—often I was too tired to make the effort.

'I had put on about two stone because of the steroids (an increase of some 20 per cent in my normal body weight) and my face had become very puffy—the typical 'moonface'. I had also developed a fungal infection on my foot and groin. I suffered from terrible mood swings and had trouble sleeping, and pernicious anaemia had also been diagnosed., Then I saw a newspaper article about Aloe Vera Gel drinking juice and started taking it a month later. For the first few weeks I felt strange (headaches and so on), but you often get that when your body is detoxifying. After that I started to feel better. Six weeks after starting on the Aloe Vera Gel I went into hospital to have a colonoscopy, to see when (not if) I would have surgery. My consultant was surprised but pleased to inform me that I was so much improved that I no longer needed it.

'I very slowly cut down my steroids until I was off them completely, and I gradually lost the puffiness and excess weight. When I saw my specialist after six months he was amazed at the improvement in my condition and asked to be sent information on what I had been taking.

'I used to have flare-ups at least once a week, but since I have been on the Aloe Vera Gel this has been reduced to one or two during periods of stress. I am now feeling considerably better than I have done for seven years and I am able once again to enjoy things I have not been able to do for years.

'My incredible recovery and continuing improvement—I call it a miracle—is due to taking aloe vera. I do, however, have a word of caution for any fellow ulcerative colitis sufferers or anyone with Crohn's who wants to try this remedy: make sure the aloe vera you buy is of the highest purity and quality. There are many brands on the market (I bought some from a health food shop and it was just like water and had no benefit at all). I have written to the National Association for Colitis and Crohn's Disease to tell them how aloe vera has changed my life—hopefully my story may help the thousands of fellow sufferers out there.

'Finally, I would like to say to anyone who has a serious condition like mine, aloe vera is not a cure but it could improve the quality of your life enormously. Talk to your doctor and/ or specialist and tell them that you want to try aloe vera, and keep them updated. If you want to write to me you can do so through The Aloe Vera Centre—the address is at the back of this book.'

William is a young man who was diagnosed HIV positive more than three years ago. At first he seemed to fall prey to colds and flu and generally felt low in spirit, and he was prescribed antibiotics on several occasions. These made him quite sick, and he felt uneasy taking so many. Then came a change for the better:

'I discovered aloe vera through a friend who invited me along to a talk. At the time I hadn't any money so I didn't buy anything. Very soon after that I fell sick again with a chest and sinus infection. Because of my condition, I also have bad problems with my gums, skin irritations and fungal infections, but worst of all, I would wake up with a sickly stomach that made me start my day feeling worried and of course sick! One thing that stuck in my mind from the party was to heal from the inside out, so I decided to really give this aloe vera stuff a go.

'I started first with Aloe Toothgel which automatically seemed to even out the acidity in my mouth and removed a lot of the yellow fur from my tongue, and my gums have been fine ever since. I have since discovered I need to use a fluoride rinse along with the toothgel and now my mouth is at its most settled.

'Soon after starting taking the drinking gel I began to notice that if I took it first thing in the morning, twenty minutes or so after waking up, my morning sickness was becoming treatable. I also found that it helped me empty my bowels in a more comfortable and complete way. I'm now able to control my bowel movements, so I can at least feel assured and have no fear of accidents through diarrhoea—unfortunately in the past I had had some mishaps which, as you can imagine, made me feel awful.

'The Aloe Vera Gelly tube has a multiplicity of uses. Before aloe vera I had problems with thrush. Applying the Gelly to my penis has stopped the red blotches from forming. I also use it between my toes, it soothes a sore bottom from too much wiping, haemorrhoids, sore nipples and it also sealed a small cut on my finger, totally stopping any bleeding (this could have become a scary experience).

'I could go on and on about incidents where I've been amazed at aloe vera's uses; it has brought me relief and a healthy mind. My energy level is much higher, enabling me to swim and be much more active, thereby improving my lifestyle. Aloe vera allows small irritations and problems to remain small. I had not had any courses of antibiotics since I started on it, and, very importantly, my T cell count is up by 100 (which can be medically explained). The choice to go with aloe vera is the one thing that has changed my life.

'It has been quite difficult actually to put these ailments on paper, as it really made me sit and think about my situation which I very rarely do, but I decided that if anyone out there gets half the relief that I have had from aloe vera, then it is worth it.'

Enid's holiday abroad was nearly ruined by a silly accident:

'On the first day, someone trod on my foot and I lost most of the nail off my big toe. As you can imagine, this was very painful and I was worried my holiday would be spoilt as I couldn't wear any of my shoes. Immediately I covered the area with Aloe Vera Gelly and a pad and bandage and didn't touch it for 24 hours.

'The next evening it was well on the way to healing and within a couple of days and several more applications of Aloe Vera Gelly it was no longer sore to touch—my holiday was saved.'

Margaret is an IBS sufferer and had been taking aloe vera regularly until her brother's unexpected death made her forget all about it.

'We shared the same house and for many weeks I was in shock and not eating. However, I have gradually started to pick up the pieces and returned to eating better, but no doubt due to all the stress the IBS returned with a vengeance.

'Strange as it may seem I forgot all about the Aloe Vera Gel until I started using the fridge again and suddenly spotted it just over a week ago. I promptly started back again on it and the results have been fantastic. My IBS seems to have eased off and I am now eating a greater variety and better.

'Another benefit which has occurred is the improvement in the condition of my skin. I had started to get small painful boils outside and inside my nose—something I had never had before. These, thankfully, have completely gone, leaving my skin soft and clear. I really do feel so very much better in such a short space of time and I am now not as depressed as I have been.'

*　　*　　*

One Christmas Heather's mother accidentally tipped a pan of boiling hot fat over her hand. She was immediately taken to accident and emergency where she was given pain-killers and a dressing was put on her hand. She was to return in three days, for at the time the burn did not look very serious. When she returned to get the dressing changed she was shocked to see how bad the burn was looking—it covered two thirds of her hand. She could not bend her fingers and there were huge blisters all over it. Again she was told to return in three days. By this time the blisters were gone but the skin was very badly cracked and looked even worse than before. The doctors told her that it would take approximately five months for her hand to heal properly. This was when Heather stepped in:

'The next day I gave her some Aloe Propolis cream. She used this two to three times a day and occasionally put Aloe Vera Gel (the drink) on the wound before applying the propolis cream. Five days later she had the bandages off and was washing dishes with detergent. The wound was completely healed except for a slight pink tinge to the affected area. My family were so amazed that we wished we had taken "before and after" pictures to show the difference.'

Frances woke up one Saturday morning with inflamed eyes and throughout the day things became gradually worse. Being a very busy mum she had little time to think about it, but by the evening, too late to get to a chemist, it was obvious that she had quite a severe bout of conjunctivitis. 'I was in a lot of discomfort' she remembers, 'and couldn't see a thing as I had to take my contact lenses out (without them I am as blind as a bat!) and I never wear glasses. I was very concerned on two counts: firstly it is extremely contagious and I didn't want to infect the rest of my family; secondly, I was in so much pain and I really needed something to help quickly.

'I remembered a good friend of mine telling me only the week before that her husband had used an aloe vera product to help cure his conjunctivitis, so I phoned her. Luckily she had some of the "magical" Aloe Activator, so my husband went round and picked up the product and I used it immediately, diluted on a one-to-one basis with boiled, filtered water. Within half an hour the pain and inflammation had been reduced. I rinsed my eyes again before I went to bed and when I woke up in the morning my eyes were totally clear, no pain, no inflammation and none of that awful yellow 'gunk'. I rinsed my eyes once again for good measure and put my contact lenses back in—without any problems.'

Having had his nose broken several times during the course of his rugby career, Brian has become quite prone to sinus and ear problems. Six years ago, while in the Middle East on holiday, he contracted a severe ear infection which spread to his sinuses, and over the next three years he was on various medications, including numerous courses of antibiotics and nasal sprays. Nothing seemed to work. He had a CAT scan and it was then suggested that he should have his sinuses drained. That didn't work the first time and had to be repeated: by now he was becoming desperate.

'It was nearly three years since I had contracted the original infection and I continued to suffer from severe pain, headaches and general discomfort in the sinus area. My sinuses became blocked very easily and were almost impossible to clear. What's more, it was very debilitating and I could not really see an end to the problem.

'Soon after this a friend introduced me to aloe vera and said there was a particular product you could use for ear, nose and throat problems. As you can imagine I was extremely reticent about spraying some plant juice up my nose! Well, all I can say is that nearly three years later I am very glad I did. The pain and discomfort went within days and I have not had any real problems since. I have drunk Aloe Vera Gel every day since and I only need to use Aloe Activator very occasionally, probably only once or twice a year.

'I have not had a cold, flu, a sore throat or any ear or sinus problems for nearly three years and, guess what—I have not had any antibiotics in that time either.'

Like Brian, Bob is now paying the price for his participation in the game of rugby:

'I am now 74 and have suffered from chronic back and neck problems for nearly twenty years as a result of injuries sustained from playing at the highest level. Having had to hang up my boots before the age of thirty, I pursued my business career in hot climates. It was not until I retired twenty years ago and came back to live in a cooler and damper climate (Scotland) that the damage I had sustained playing rugby began to take its toll. I quickly began to suffer from neck and back problems and very soon became a regular visitor to both chiropractors and osteopaths.

'About eighteen months ago someone told me that drinking aloe vera might help my condition. I decided to try it and after a few months I certainly felt better. I just carried on taking the drink and thought no more of it until my wife remarked that for the first time in about nineteen years I hadn't had any arthritic pains in my back or neck and hadn't felt the need to visit the chiropractor or osteopath.

'The only thing that had changed in my diet was the aloe vera, so I would thoroughly recommend it to anyone with similar problems. It also seems to boost one's energy levels and certainly helps the digestive system.'

Stella had suffered over a long period of time from fatigue, along with frequent headaches, stomach pains and bloating. She also had skin allergies which had plagued her for a few years and had sought numerous solutions and taken various medications, without relief. Then a friend recommended Aloe Vera Juice, and within a short time Stella was reporting a noticeable improvement:

'I have been taking the juice for about six weeks now, and genuinely feel a lot less tired and consequently a lot more active as a result of my increased energy level. My skin is also looking slightly better and seems to be healing a lot quicker, and the bloating and headaches have decreased.

'I have been very encouraged by these results and have started to use Aloe Vera Rejuvenating Gel on my skin, which I have found to be very calming and healing. My mother has now also started to take the juice as she was so impressed with my improvements. She too has been feeling a lot less tired, her sleeping patterns have improved and she no longer takes her diuretic tablets, which she has relied on for many years.'

'For 25 years,' reports Juliet, 'I have suffered from migraine, PMS, thrush and irritable bowel syndrome (IBS). My joints and stomach were painful and swollen. I was overweight and looked six months pregnant, my chest wheezed and I felt permanently tired as my sleep was disturbed by aches and pains. Even after a "good" night's rest I still felt tired and would fall asleep even in the middle of town if I stopped for a rest.

'After years of prescriptions for various drugs, like aspirin and cortisone for pain, hormones for PMS and antifungals for thrush, I felt very ill and developed ulcers to add to the misery. I became very disillusioned with these treatments and totally fed up with being constantly ill.

'I started to learn about alternative therapies and to practise yoga. I slowly improved my diet, cutting out red meat, tea, coffee and sugar, for example, and eating more wholefoods and vitamin supplements. This was very difficult, especially if, like me, you are a chocaholic. Although I improved, I felt I could be a lot better.

'After a particularly bad attack of candida and IBS, I contacted a therapist who specialised in food allergies and colonic irrigation. She explained that the toxins in my system needed to be cleared out. Apparently I was allergic to wheat and yeast, foods that I had been eating for many years, which were actually making me ill. She advised me to tale Aloe Vera Juice and vitamins.

'I have been taking aloe vera for the past eight months and feel so well I cannot believe it. I have lost two stone in weight and no longer suffer with PMS and migraines. My friends can see the difference, and I can now stay awake all day and sleep at night. I am even learning to swim, something I thought I would never be able to do. Although it was not easy to change my diet, it has made the most amazing difference to my life. So I will stick with it and keep taking the Aloe Vera.'

When Mary was first advised that aloe vera might help her ME she was going through a remission period. As these had become longer and longer and her relapses shorter and shorter although incredibly painful, she did not think she needed any help: she was perfectly happy with the way she was feeling in comparison with how dreadful she had felt before. She therefore tried Aloe Vera Juice, women's multivitamins and Super Bee tablets with some scepticism, having already spent a fortune on many other remedies which proved useless. However, she very soon noticed a change.

'On day two I had the most horrendous headaches which lasted three days, which did not worry me unduly as I knew this was a process of detoxifying. On day five I woke up for the first time for seven years naturally at 7.30 a.m. and actually felt like getting out of bed. Over the next few days I noticed a remarkable improvement in my eyesight, clearness of thinking and capacity for work.

'Since then I have had endless compliments on the change in me; my hair has grown thicker and my skin has become incredibly clear and healthy. I am still taking four capfuls twice a day with two women's multivitamins and two Super Bee tablets and would not dream of stopping, although I feel wonderful, as one weekend I forgot to take the juice away with me and within twelve hours all the pains had started to come back.

'However, I would like to pass on one word of warning: whatever you do, do not overdo it because you will naturally exhaust yourself with the amazing new-found energy which, in my case, I had not had for over seven years.

'This has really been a new lease of life for me and I am eternally grateful.'

George too was sceptical when he first heard about the claims made for aloe vera:

'At the time I was suffering considerably from the effects of a duodenal ulcer. Since orthodox medicine had failed to give any relief, and being of the mind to 'try anything', I decided to give the Aloe Juice a try. Not only have I had no recurrence of the ulcer pain, I was surprised to note that the severe arthritis within my right elbow had virtually disappeared!

'I believe that the rapid healing of the wound after a hernia operation was also due to this product and I now have a feeling of overall improved good health.'

CHAPTER 7

How To Use
Aloe Vera

Obviously, aloe vera is not a panacea for all ills, and because
it is a natural substance, like herbs for instance, it can take
longer to have a beneficial effect on some chronic symptoms
than a chemically-based drug. This is because it works
harmoniously with the body's own self-regulating systems
rather than overcoming them and leaving them in a depleted
state.

For example, it is now well known that a course of antibiotics can so successfully override (rather than gently boost)
the immune system, killing off both the 'good' and the 'bad'
bacteria in the digestive tract, that it can take up to six weeks
for the 'good' flora to re-establish itself and continue its job
of protecting the body against infection.

The following hints and tips are therefore intended to
help first-time users of aloe vera get the most benefit from
it.

1   Give aloe vera enough time to work—at least three
    months—so that your body has time to adjust to this
    'softly, softly' approach.
2   Get good advice from someone who knows about aloe
    vera and how it works.

3   When you start taking aloe vera as a drink you need to
     establish what dosage is right for you. At first you could
     try as little as a teaspoon at a time, or a dessertspoon or
     a tablespoon, depending on how you feel each day. After
     a day or so you might want to take another (perhaps one
     before breakfast, and one at night). If that feels all right
     you may want to try increasing the dosage to between
     two and four tablespoons per day (the average daily dose
     for an adult).

     The dosage depends on whether you are taking it just
     as a tonic (I take two small wine glasses per day as a
     tonic—it seems to boost my energy levels and has helped
     me remain free of colds and various other bugs for the
     last three years) or for a more pressing concern such as
     a digestive or skin problem. You might find it most ben-
     eficial to take it little and often throughout the day, but
     others might prefer to take it in one or two large doses.

4   Most people take it on an empty stomach, but some say
     it aids digestion when taken just before or after a heavy
     meal. You could try both in an emergency!

     While we are on the subject of digestion, this might
     be a good time to discuss a difficult subject—detox-
     ification. This process of 'all the bad stuff coming
     out' can and does happen with the use of aloe vera.
     One of its properties is that of a cleanser and purifier. It
     does not necessarily happen with everybody, but there
     are tell-tale signs such as unexplained skin rashes, head-
     aches, puffy skin, wind, tiredness, queasiness, aches and
     pains.

     If you have a chronic condition like, for example, ME,
     IBS or arthritis, you might find a temporary worsening
     of symptoms as part of this detoxifying process. Which
     leads us to the next tip.

5   If any symptoms arise for no apparent reason and you
     think the cause might be the aloe vera:
     a   don't panic;

b   ask your adviser;
c   take his or her advice!

If there is no one to ask, you should stop taking the aloe vera for a couple of days or until the symptoms disappear. Then start on a very low dose and gradually build up again.

Or you can phone The Aloe Vera Centre for advice on their Helpline Number: 0181-871-5205, or leave a message on the Helpline Answerphone.

You might find you don't need quite as much as before, or you might need to take it at a different time of the day, or you might need to take more for a while. Give your body time to adjust.

6   Remember to keep opened bottles of the aloe vera drinking gel or juice IN THE FRIDGE.

7   If you want to travel with it, don't decant it into another bottle and stash it in your hand luggage. Take the proper bottle, safely tucked between two ice-packs, in a small 'cooler bag' (and make sure you put the container in a fridge before the ice-packs have melted).

8   Babies and young children could start with one or two teaspoons a day, gradually increasing the number until the right level is found.

9   If you have an allergy or skin problems, it is a good idea to do a patch test first of either the drink or the lotion you want to use.

10   Remember to ensure that a wound, particularly a puncture wound, is thoroughly cleansed before applying aloe vera. Because of its ability to penetrate deeply into the skin it could carry particles of dirt down with it.

11   Aloe vera is non-toxic and is safe to use alongside conventional methods of medication.

12   Diarrhoea, as a part of the detoxification of the body, is only a problem if it lasts longer than a couple of days. Drink plenty of filtered water every day and lower the dose of aloe vera.

13 Constipation can be improved by drinking more aloe vera until the bowel is working comfortably again. Again, drinking plenty of filtered water can help.

SAFETY FIRST AND LAST

If you are at all unsure about embarking on a course of any natural remedy, including aloe vera, consult a doctor or a nutritionist first. Reputable companies have a doctor and other health professionals on their advisory boards, who are generally available for advice through the company's own trained distributors. You should also remember that not all doctors will be aware of the potential benefits of aloe vera; many of them haven't even heard of it. My GP, who is a young Chinese doctor, was very positive (something of an exception at the present time) when I told him that I took aloe vera as a tonic and detoxifier.

Pregnant Women

In the past pregnant women have generally been advised not to take aloe vera internally because it was reputed to cause bowel spasms. This is partly true but only relates to those products which may contain the purgative substance, known as aloin, which can cause this to happen. The leading aloe vera products only use the inner leaf gel, and if it has been properly stabilised and processed it will not contain aloin. I have met many pregnant women in the past few years who have taken aloe vera as a tonic or health drink or to help with problems like constipation, tiredness and so on. They have not only found aloe vera to be extremely beneficial in terms of increased energy, but have also found it helps with any digestive problems.

Aloe vera contains not only a host of vitamins, minerals, amino acids, enzymes and polysaccharides, it also contains folic acid which has been found to be highly beneficial for pregnant women. It is now scientifically claimed that taking folic acid can help reduce the risk of spina bifida in babies. The quality of the aloe vera you drink is the key factor in whether or not it will benefit you.

Diabetics

In some people it has been discovered that drinking aloe vera can increase the amount of insulin produced by the body. People with diabetes must therefore be monitored closely by their doctor, as some people have found that the amount of insulin prescribed can be reduced.

Any Contra-indications?

No, not to our knowledge, as aloe vera is a non-toxic substance. It is always wise to do a patch test first, as stated previously, if you are susceptible to allergic reactions. Always take advice when using it internally, especially for the treatment of wounds, eyes, sinuses and ears. Water it down with filtered water only, when required.

BODY ROUTE MAP—PRODUCT INDEX

A—eyes, nose, throat, ears: conjunctivitis, sinusitis, infections.
PRODUCT: Aloe activator (aloe spray can be used in the nose for infections).

B—scalp: eczema, psoriasis, hair loss, dryness, itchiness.
PRODUCT: aloe vera gelly.

C—hair: hair loss, lacklustre hair, dandruff.
PRODUCT: aloe jojoba shampoo, aloe jojoba conditioner.

D—teeth, gums: gingivitis, receding/bleeding gums, mouth ulcers.
PRODUCT: aloe toothgel, aloe vera gelly.

E—lips: chapped, cracked lips, cold sores.
PRODUCT: aloe lip salve.

F—face: acne, dry skin, psoriasis.
PRODUCT: aloe vera gelly, aloe lotion, aloe moisturising lotion, aloe propolis cream, plus a complete skin nutrition range including cleanser, toner, face mask, day cream and night cream.

G—neck, shoulders: all muscles, strain, stiffness.
PRODUCT: aloe heat lotion, aloe lotion.

H—underarms: perspiration, odour.
PRODUCT: aloe deodorant.

I—skin (all over): for dry skin or general skin disorders.
PRODUCT: aloe liquid soap, aloe bath gelee, aloe moisturising lotion, aloe propolis cream, aloe vera gelly.

J—skin (all over): exfoliating and sloughing off dead skin cells.
PRODUCT: aloe vera face and body scrub, aloe vera bath gelee (with loofah).

KNOW YOUR WAY AROUND?
Where and What You Can Use Aloe Vera For—a Body Route Map

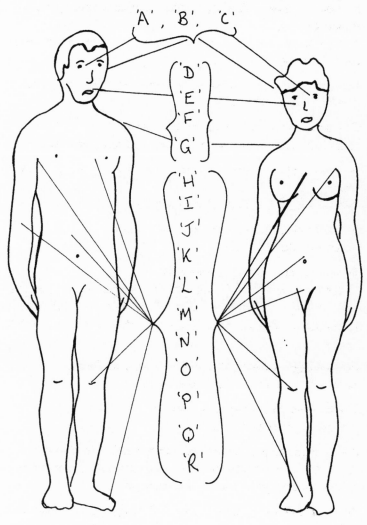

K—entire digestive system.
PRODUCT: aloe vera drinking gels and juices.

L—fingers, knees and all joints: arthritis, gout, etc.
PRODUCT: Aloe vera drinking gels and juices, aloe heat lotion.

M—back: pain.
PRODUCT: aloe vera drinking gels and juices, aloe heat lotion.

N—feet, toes, heels.
PRODUCT: aloe vera gelly, aloe propolis cream, aloe lotion.

O—general health tonic and detoxification.
PRODUCT: aloe vera drinking gels and juices.

P—breathing: difficulties associated with asthma and other lung disorders.
PRODUCT: aloe vera drinking gels and juices.

Q—renal and urinary tract system: cystitis, etc.
PRODUCT: aloe vera juice with cranberries.

R—genital organs: thrush, candida.
PRODUCT: aloe vera gelly, aloe vera drinking gels and juices.

THE A to Z OF REMEDIES

What Aloe Vera Has Been Used for Over the Years

Historically, we find that aloe vera has been used to treat a wide range of ailments and disorders in both humans and animals, and many more uses for the leaf gel have been suggested over the years.

A
Abrasions, abscesses, acidity, acne, allergic reactions, allergies, anaemia, arthritis, asthma, athlete's foot.
B
Bad breath, baldness, blisters, boils, bronchitis, bruises, burns, bursitis.
C
Candida, canker sores, carbuncles, cataracts, chapped skin, cold sores, colds, colic, colitis, conjunctivitis, contusions, coughs, cradle cap, cuts (lacerations), cystitis.
D
Dandruff, denture sores, depression, dermatitis, diabetes, dry skin, duodenal ulcers, dysentry.
E
Eczema, epidermitis.
F
Fever blisters, fissured nipples.
G
Gastritis, genital herpes, gingivitis, glands (swollen), glaucoma.
H
Haemorrhoids, headaches, heat rash, hepatitis, herpes.
I
IBS, impetigo, indigestion, inflamed joints and skin, ingrown toenails, insomnia.
J
Jaundice.

K
Keratosis.
L
Laryngitis, leg ulcers, lupus.
M
Mastitis in dairy cattle, ME, menopausal flushes, mouth ulcers, MS, muscle cramp/strains.
N
Nappy rash, nausea.
O
Oedema, oral disorders.
P
Peptic ulcers, pin worms, PMT, poison ivy/oak, prickly heat, prostatitis, psoriasis.
R
Radiation burns, razor burns, ringworm.
S
Seborrhea, shingles, skin sores, sore throat, sprains, stings, stretch marks, styes, sunburn.
T
Tendonitis, thrush, tonsilitis, trachoma, tuberculosis.
U
Ulcerations of all kinds, ulcerative colitis, urticaria.
V
Vaginitis, varicose veins, venereal sores, vulvitis.
W
Wind burns, wounds of all kinds (surface).
X, Y, Z
X-ray burns, yeast infections.

This is by no means a totally exhaustive summary of all the ailments and disorders for which aloe vera products can be used. We have tried to give you examples of the more common problems and disorders experienced by those people we have spoken to.

If you or anyone you know has an interesting case history you would like to share with us (anonymity guaranteed), please contact me, Alasdair Barcroft, by writing to me c/o the publishers. We may be able to consider your story for any future editions of the book.

CHAPTER 8

Animal Magic

Aloe vera has been used for hundreds of years by farmers and other animal-breeders in countries where the plant grows indigenously. For example, they would wrap the sliced leaves around a wounded animal's leg, as a splint or a poultice, and allow the gel to do its work, reducing swelling, fighting infection, healing flesh and skin. Only in the last thirty years have clinical studies been carried out to verify and expand this traditional knowledge and practice.

In their book *Creatures in Our Care—The Veterinary Uses of Aloe Vera*, Bill Coats, RPh, and Richard E. Holland, DVM, describe in detail how aloe vera can be used in the treatment of numerous internal and external disorders, as well as in the healing of wounds, from surface abrasions to quite deep puncture wounds. All animals can be treated, from small wild animals and birds to cats and dogs, up to the large animals like horses and cattle.

More and more veterinary surgeons in the UK are now becoming interested in stabilised aloe vera and are using it on their patients. Some time ago my wife sold several products to a great friend of ours to use on her twelve horses. This friend was amazed, when she next saw her vet (from one of the leading equine practices in the UK) to find that he also used some of the same products. Quite an endorsement! Our friend uses a range of topical products as well as aloe vera drink (the same as humans take) to help with listlessness and lethargy in some of her horses. She feels it gives them more energy and helps boost their immune system.

Many other people who keep or are involved with animals are now beginning to realise how effective aloe vera can be as a healer, both internally and externally. One unsung heroine of wildlife rescue in Sussex uses aloe vera as part of her treatment for wild creatures:

'I've used it on everything from crow's feet (literally!) to a hedgehog's nose. The crow was a teenager which was brought in with very sore feet. I treated them with Aloe Propolis cream every day for a week until they healed. A large chicken with a bad leg developed sores on her bottom from having to lie down all the time. I applied Aloe Vera Gelly which soothed them and they healed up.

'A female thrush had been attacked by a cat and had a lacerated and broken wing. I doused it well with Aloe Veterinary spray, then put the Aloe Vera Gelly on it before the wing was strapped up. It healed well and the bird was subsequently released.

'I've treated two of my six dogs with aloe vera, both of them Golden Retrievers. I used Aloe Vera Lotion and the Gelly on some eczema patches which healed up quickly and the same products were used to treat a very sore front paw on the other dog.

'A collared dove was rescued from the jaws of a dog. The bird's leg was broken and it had several wounds all over its body. The vet set the leg but a swelling developed below the splint, so I applied Aloe Vera Gelly above and below the splint. Gradually the swelling went down and when the splint was eventually removed the leg was fine and had healed well.

'A jackdaw had been attacked by magpies and had sustained a terrible throat wound, and another on top of its wing. I treated it with Aloe Vera Lotion and the Aloe Vera Gelly and the wounds healed beautifully, and several weeks later I released the bird back into the wild.

'A hen pheasant was hit by a car and almost scalped, with a hole in the top of her head and a nasty wound in her neck. I used Aloe Propolis cream for all these wounds. They healed well, and she was released a few weeks later, having been courted by a wild paramour from the other side of her cage whenever she was out in the garden!

'A large white goose was badly mauled by a fox and had to have one wing amputated. The stump developed a nasty sore, so I treated it with Aloe Propolis cream and it worked very well.

'I have noticed that the Aloe Propolis is particularly useful for treating birds. It sinks into the skin so quickly and completely, with no stickiness at all, that it doesn't matter if it gets onto the feathers because it won't clog them up.

'A rabbit was hit by a car and had a badly damaged eye. I bathed it with a weak solution of Aloe Activator and lukewarm purified water. It worked: the eye healed quickly and the rabbit went back to the wild to do what rabbits do best!

'Then there was the hedgehog, a baby, weighing only two ounces, whose nose had been chewed by a cat. It couldn't suck and breathe at the same time. When I fed it from a dropper, it would take alternate sips and breaths. I applied the Aloe Vera Gelly on its nose every day and it healed beautifully. The hedgehog grew to a strapping one-and-a-half pounds and was released.

'Sometimes I have to treat myself for bites, scratches and other accidents. A tawny owl was startled by something as I was holding it against my chest with one hand and opening its cage door with the other. It dug its claws into my jumper, my blouse and my thermal vest, right through to my skin. Owls' claws are hooked and very sharp, and the birds are tenacious and very strong. I had a punctured left breast. It was extremely sore and had drawn blood. Aloe Propolis cream soothed and healed it very quickly.

'Although the Aloe Veterinary spray is formulated with animals in mind, I must say that it worked wonders for me when I had a nasty bite from one of my parrots on my forearm. Parrots being meat eaters with ferocious beaks, their bite wounds usually require tetanus jabs (which I have as routine, anyway, just in case), as infection usually sets in and can be very nasty. The nearest thing to hand was the Aloe Veterinary spray which I sprayed on. I applied Aloe Propolis cream for the next couple of days and then forgot about it. And I'm still alive to tell the tale!'

*   *   *

Many pet-owners use aloe vera products to treat wounds and ailments. The following are just a few examples from many accounts of cats and dogs that have benefited from this healing plant.

A RETRIEVER WITH INFECTED EARS

'My retriever had the beginnings of an ear infection to which he is rather prone when he has been swimming in a stagnant pond in the woods. I put two drops of Aloe Activator in each ear and also used it to bathe and clean the outer ears. Within minutes I could tell that he was much more comfortable and he stopped scratching at them. After two more treatments within the following 24 hours he was completely cured. I now use the Activator routinely as an ear wash.'

A HEALTH TONIC FOR AN ELDERLY CAT

'About eighteen months ago my seventeen-year-old neutered tom had a stroke, plus two "aftershocks". This was before I knew about aloe vera, and he was treated by a vet. "Cadbury Cat" recovered slowly although he is rather lopsided and falls off things.

'Six months ago I noticed he was looking rather scraggy
and his coat was a little "stary". He refuses to eat food which
he regards as having been doctored with vitamin powder, so
I mixed in a half a teaspoon of Aloe Vera Gel drink and
managed to go up to three-quarters of a teaspoon in each of
his twice-daily meals. Within days he was looking brighter
and within a fortnight he had gained weight and had the sheen
back on his coat. He was on aloe vera for about six weeks,
and today he is still fit and ready for a game. He even caught
a mouse last week.'

A RETRIEVER'S CHEST WOUND

'He had been leaping about through the woods on his walk,
and when we got home I saw blood dripping from a deep,
open wound over his ribcage. It was a gaping cut about an
inch long and more than a quarter of an inch across the middle.
I washed the wound thoroughly with Aloe Vera Soap, packed
it with Aloe Vera Gelly and stuck a large plaster over it,
repeating this four times in the first day. The next day I used
Aloe Activator, which is 99.6 per cent pure aloe vera liquid,
to clean the wound instead of the soap, and repeated the pack-
ing with Aloe Vera Gelly and covered it with plaster.

'Over the next two days he was kept on the lead for his
daily walk so that the wound could remain clean and dry. On
the third day the cushions of flesh were beginning to close
together—the "floor" moving up and the two side-cushions
meeting. A soft, pliant scab formed, leaving a small drainage
hole in the centre which would "weep" a lot of clear fluid
every day or so. It was always odour-free, and although the
immediate area surrounding the wound was hot and swollen,
the wound itself was pink and clean. It was obvious that there
was no infection.

'The dog enjoyed the four-times-a-day ritual and would roll
on to his back at the first sight of the aloe vera tube, with a
huge grin on his face. Every day the wound shrank and by the

tenth day the scab had hardened and formed a narrow 'frill', rather like the ridge of pastry on a Cornish pasty!'

A CANINE SUCCESS

'Although I bought Aloe Vera Gel drink for my own use, I am also finding that it is proving very successful for one of our Irish Setter dogs. For some years he has had problems with an enlarged spleen and hiatus hernia, which causes him to retch, bringing up bile or mucus. In spite of using Tegamet syrup the problem has become increasingly bad. On the off-chance we gave him some gel, since when he has only retched once instead of three or four times a night. Before this we were beginning to think we would shortly have to put him to sleep. Incidentally, aloe vera continues to help me with my tummy problem, too!'

A SKIN ALLERGY

'For several years my collie-cross dog has suffered from a pollen allergy in the spring and summer. Up until now the only effective treatment has been steroids which have had the side-effect of weight gain and excessive thirst. I now use the Aloe Veterinary spray on the irritated areas and have managed to cut the steroids down to a quarter of a tablet per day. He had a particularly sore patch on his elbow which responded well to the aloe vera spray and soon healed up.'

Many more people with animals tell of different aloe vera products they have used to help treat and heal a wide spectrum of ailments and disorders, from eczema (Westies seem particularly prone to this problem) to arthritis, colitis and other digestive disorders. Anyone wanting to know more about aloe vera and animals can contact The Aloe Vera Centre (see Appendix 1). Below is a listing of the sort of ailments that aloe vera may help, and some recommendations of the different products that can be used.

ALOE VERA AND ITS USE IN COMMON ANIMAL AILMENTS

Abrasions: aloe vera gelly, aloe veterinary spray.

Abscesses: aloe activator, aloe veterinary spray.

Arthritis: aloe vera gel drink, aloe heat lotion on joints.

Bites: aloe spray, aloe vera gelly, aloe veterinary spray.

Blood in urine: aloe vera juice with cranberries.

Bruises: aloe heat lotion, aloe vera gelly, aloe activator.

Burns: aloe vera gelly, aloe veterinary spray.

Catarrh: aloe activator (2 or 3 squirts up nostrils 3 times daily).

Conjunctivitis: aloe activator.

Convalescence: aloe vera gel drink (100g (4oz) daily).

Coronet injuries: aloe activator, aloe veterinary spray, aloe spray, aloe vera gelly.

Cough: aloe activator, aloe vera gelly (down throat several times a day).

Cuts: aloe activator, aloe vera gelly, aloe vera gel drink.

Diarrhoea: aloe vera gel drink.

Eye injuries: aloe activator.

Inflammation: aloe activator or aloe veterinary spray followed by aloe heat lotion, aloe vera gel drink.

Laminitis: aloe vera gel drink.

Limestone infection: aloe activator, aloe lotion, aloe heat lotion, aloe vera gel drink.

Mud fever: aloe veterinary spray, aloe activator, aloe propolis cream.

Nasal discharge: aloe activator (2 or 3 squirts up nostrils 3 times daily.

Pain and swelling: aloe vera gel drink, aloe activator, aloe vera gelly, aloe veterinary spray, aloe spray.

Pharyngitis: aloe activator.

Puncture wounds: Clean with aloe activator, pack with aloe vera gelly, aloe propolis cream, aloe veterinary spray.

Rashes: aloe spray, aloe vera gelly, aloe veterinary spray.

Respiratory problems: aloe activator, aloe vera gelly.

Sarcoids/Proud flesh: aloe vera gelly.

Skin disorders (eczema, ringworm): aloe veterinary spray, aloe lotion, aloe vera gelly, aloe propolis cream.

Sore legs: aloe heat lotion, aloe vera gelly, aloe activator.

Sore mouth: aloe vera gelly.

Sore throat: aloe activator, aloe vera gelly.

Sprains and strains: aloe activator or aloe veterinary spray followed by aloe heat lotion, aloe vera gel drink.

Strangles: aloe vera gel drink (approx. 100g (4oz) in feed or water daily). Combine 50g (2oz) aloe vera gelly and aloe activator and squirt down throat daily.

Sunburn: aloe spray, aloe vera gelly, aloe veterinary spray.

Suspensory ligament: aloe activator, aloe heat lotion, aloe veterinary spray.

Sweet itch: aloe vera gelly, aloe propolis cream.

Swelling: aloe vera gel drink, aloe activator, aloe vera gelly, aloe veterinary spray, aloe spray.

Swollen joints: aloe heat lotion, aloe vera gel drink, aloe veterinary spray.

Throat infections: Combine 50g (2oz) aloe activator and aloe vera gelly and squirt down throat twice daily.

Thrush: Clean with hydrogen peroxide and pack with aloe vera gelly.

Uterine infections: aloe activator, aloe veterinary spray.

Virus: aloe vera gel drink (100g (4 oz) daily).

Warts: Rub in aloe vera gelly several times a day.

Wounds: For minor ones apply aloe veterinary lotion. For severe ones cleanse with aloe activator and pack with aloe vera gelly.

NOTE: Wash pets' blankets or cushions and horses' rugs, tack and numnahs with aloe detergent. Also good for sponging mats under feeding bowls of cats and dogs.

CHAPTER 9

Last Thoughts

I hope that this book has given you an insight into one of nature's most remarkable plants, its history and why it is only now, as we approach the end of another millennium, that aloe vera is making a well-deserved come-back. It is undoubtedly proving to be one of nature's great healers and is at last beginning to overturn the often ill-founded prejudices that seem to have surrounded it in the last few centuries. I have tried to encapsulate as much useful information as I could without making the book a scientific tome. I hope it has been easy to read and, indeed, to understand, and that you can see the wide range of benefits that aloe vera can give us, whether taken internally as a drink or applied topically, or both.

When I set out to write this book I had not intended it to be a crusade on any particular aspect, but rather an introduction to one of nature's miracles and the significant health role it can play in a world where good nutrition and a healthy diet are often sacrificed on the altar of convenience as we all rush around fulfilling business or personal commitments, eating ready-made meals 'on the run'.

However, it would be remiss of me, even irresponsible, if I did not take this opportunity to stress the point about the vast disparity in the quality of aloe vera products being marketed in many countries. The trend towards natural products, including aloe vera, is fast becoming a tidal wave and it is vital that the quality ethic is upheld by all those involved and especially those in the aloe vera industry. As the demand for aloe vera grows, so does the opportunity for exploitation by manufacturers who either do not meet the exacting requirements of the International Aloe Science Council or whose products simply do not contain enough aloe vera to be effective.

In researching this book I have been amazed at what I have found. Some companies, for example, are using the IASC Seal of Approval without the right to do so. You may ask, and quite rightly so, why would they want to do that? Quite simply because they know it gives them and their products more credibility and thus helps generate more sales. I would ask you to reread Chapter 3 and Appendix 1, and suggest you take careful note of what is said there. Other companies make claims about the 'strength', 'power' or 'concentration' of their products compared to others—claims which may not stand up to close scientific examination. Some companies even use 'endorsements' by industry experts without their knowledge and very often out of context.

Remember, whatever it says on the label, make sure that when you look at the percentage of aloe vera content, it is given by volume—that is, what percentage of the total contents is aloe vera. You should ensure that the main ingredient of the product you buy is '100 per cent stabilised aloe vera gel' and that aloe vera is the primary ingredient, at the top of the list of ingredients. Finally, on the subject of quality, there is no reason nowadays why you should buy any aloe vera products, be they drinks, creams, lotions or shampoos, without insisting on a 90-day money-back guarantee and/or the IASC Seal of Approval. You could also insist that the products you buy are processed from aloe vera plants that have been grown organically and do not contain any chemical preservatives.

You have a choice. It is entirely up to you what products you buy, but don't be disappointed if the one you buy doesn't do you any good. Don't blame aloe vera, blame the way it has been processed and manufactured. Price is not necessarily an indicator of quality or effectiveness – there are some very expensive aloe vera products that do not have the same amount of 'active ingredient' as some less expensive brands!

Remember, as I have said before in this book, 'you pays your money and you takes your choice'. It would be very sad indeed if aloe vera, through no fault of its own, again acquired a bad reputation. I personally do not think that will happen because there are organisations like the IASC, there are reputable growers and manufacturers and there are bodies in several countries like The Aloe Vera Centre in London, which provide advice on how and when to use aloe vera.

As far as I am concerned, aloe vera has become an integral part of my daily health and diet regime. You should try it too—it could do you a power of good!

How does one summarise more than three thousand years of history in the few pages of a book? How can one condense the many years of experience of therapists and other professionals and the case histories of literally thousands of people who have used aloe vera and found it beneficial? Quite simply, it's impossible! Aloe vera has so far stood the test of time, and for far longer than any man-made medicine. I hope that people will continue to write about it and that scientists will continue to try to unlock its secret mechanisms of healing.

I believe, as we go into the next millennium, that people all over the world will begin to realise, as they discover the power of aloe vera, that the legend really has come of age and that it is truly one of nature's 'miracle healers'.

Glossary

ALOIN. Purgative compound found under the rind of the leaf.

ANALGESIC. Ability to diminish pain by acting on the central nervous system.

ANTIBIOTIC. Ability to slow down or stop the development of pathogenic microbes.

ANTI-INFLAMMATORY. Ability to act against the inflammation of tissues caused by physical, chemical or biological aggression.

ASTRINGENT. Ability to tighten tissues, to stop haemorrhages, diarrhoea, etc.

BACTERICIDAL. Ability to destroy bacteria.

CATHARTIC. Ability to purify, a mild laxative.

COLLAGEN. Fibrous protein, principal constituent of the intercellular substance of conjunctive tissues.

DERMIS. Conjunctive tissue which, together with the epithelium, forms the skin.

ELIXIR. A liquid preparation usually made of aromatic vegetable substances in alcohol or wine.

EMOLLIENT. Ability to soften, e.g. skin.

ENZYMES. Proteins with great catalytic power, facilitating the metabolism of molecules produced by the genes.

FIBROBLAST. Cells of conjunctive tissue responsible for the fabrication of collagen fibres which form the skin and muscle tissues.

FUNGICIDAL. Ability to destroy pathogenic fungus causing mycosis of the skin.

HAEMOSTATIC. Substance which is coagulating and vascoconstricting, thus stops bleeding.

LAXATIVE. A substance which facilitates bowel movement and prevents or cures constipation.

METABOLISM. The biological and chemical processes which take place in the cells to transform food into energy.

VIRUCIDAL. Ability to destroy a virus.

Appendices

1 ORGANISATIONS AND USEFUL ADDRESSES

The International Aloe Science Council (IASC)
415 East Airport Freeway, Suite 365, Irving,
Texas 75062, USA.

There has been a spate of products claiming to have the International Aloe Science Council Seal of Approval and a number of products that refer, on their labels, to the IASC and bear a seal almost identical in shape and design to the IASC Seal of Approval. That has prompted us to ask some questions about the subject on behalf of you, the potential customer. Here are the answers.

Q What is the International Aloe Science Council?
A   It is an independent body, set up to monitor standards within the aloe vera industry worldwide.
Q Where is it based?
A   In Irving, Texas—a town that is part of the Dallas conurbation.
Q How is it funded?
A   The Council is funded entirely by fees received. All members pay annual membership fees, and if a member wants to have a product certified, an analysis fee is charged. Members also pay an annual certification fee for every product that has been certified.
Q Who are its members?
A   Agro-Mar Inc, Nevada;
Aloe Laboratories Inc., Texas;
El Mar Enterprises Inc., California;

Terry Laboratories Inc., Florida;

Aloe Complete Inc., California;

Aloe Vera of America, Texas (this is a Forever Living Products company);

LODC, Texas;

Univera Inc., Texas;

Aloecorp., Texas;

Aloe World Inc., Dominican Republic;

Namyang Aloe Co., Korea.

Q *What is the IASC Seal of Approval?*

A It is a certification of the quality of aloe vera products. It includes the auditing of the manufacturing facilities and processes, as well as analysis of the product itself.

Q *How do you get the IASC Seal of Approval for your products?*

A All aloe vera suppliers are invited to submit their products for certification by the IASC. If a supplier is certified and his or her products contain the specified minimum amount of aloe vera, then the company is eligible to apply for the IASC Seal of Approval.

Companies who want the right to display the seal must have their products analysed by independent experts who use approved procedures developed by the Council's Science and Technical Committee.

Q *How many other aloe products genuinely hold the Seal of Approval?*

A The IASC told us that, as of September 1996, apart from Forever Living Products, NO OTHER COMPANY selling aloe vera in the UK has its Seal of Approval on any products.

Q *What can the IASC tell us about 'whole leaf aloe'?*

A As its name implies, whole leaf aloe is made by pulping the whole of the leaf, including rind and inner gel. As this would contain the aloin which acts as a strong purgative, the pulp is then passed through a carbon filter block which absorbs the aloin, making the resulting product suitable

118

for human consumption. However, the question of which other nutrients are absorbed by the filter has not yet been fully answered.

Q   *What other definitions of aloe vera are there?*

A   **Aloe vera gel or juice** is defined as the naturally occurring, processed, undiluted (100 per cent), parenchymal tissue obtained from the *Aloe barbadensis Miller* plant, to which no more than 5 per cent additives (including preservatives) shall be added as part of the processing. An **aloe vera beverage** is defined as an ingestible product containing a minimum of 50 per cent aloe vera juice as defined in the reporting procedure adopted by the IASC. An **aloe vera drink** is defined similarly to the beverage, but the minimum content of aloe is only 10 per cent. In addition, there are definitions for aloe vera spray dried, freeze dried, concentrate, pulp and oil.

The Institute for Optimum Nutrition (ION)

The Institute for Optimum Nutrition offers personal consultations with qualified nutritionists, including a one-day Optimum Nutrition Workshop, Homestudy Course and the Nutrition Consultants Diploma Course. It also offers the *CNEAT Directory of Nutrition Consultants* to help you find a nutrition consultant in your area. For details of courses, consultations or publications and a free information pack, send an A5 SAE to:

ION, Blades Court, Deodar Road, London SW15 2NU, or phone 0181-877-9993.

Other Useful Names and Addresses:

The Aloe Vera Centre*
Gardiner House, 3/9 Broomhill Road, London SW18 4JQ.
Tel: 0181-871-5083/5205. Fax: 0181-871-5203. Contact: Mary
Barcroft.

Aloe Vera Research Institute
2681 Cameron Park Drive #122, Cameron Park,
CA84120, USA.

Venetia Armitage (nutritionist)
71 York Mansions, Prince of Wales Drive, London SW11
4BW. Tel: 0171-720-2984.

Adrian Blake (homoeopath)
12 Cosway Street, London NW1 5NR. Tel: 0171-224-8944.
Fax: 0171-724-5766.

Kate Ker (stress counsellor)
Brockhurst Farm, Dunsfold Road, Alfold, nr Cranleigh, Surrey
GU6 8JB. Tel: 01403-752229.

Anoosh Liddell (reflexologist and aromatherapist)
3 Vernon Road, Bushey, Watford, Herts WD2 2JL. Tel: 01923-
460036. e-mail: r@rliddell.demon.co.uk.

Rosemary Titterington (herbalist)
Iden Croft Herbs, Frittenden Road, Staplehurst, Kent TN12
ODH. Tel: 01580-891432. Fax: 01580-89241.

* 'Aloe Vera Centre Ltd.' is a registered trading name and The Aloe
Vera Centre in London is the only organisation in the UK permitted to use
'Aloe Vera Centre' in its name.

2   ALOE VERA PRODUCTS

We have listed below a range of typical aloe vera products now available in the UK.

Drinks

Aloe Vera Gel and Juice drinks: one of nature's best anti-inflammatory, detoxifying and nutritional health drinks.
Aloe Vera Juices with cranberries: the same nutritional and health benefits as the above, but with the additional healing properties of cranberries.

Skin Care

Aloe propolis creams: intensive moisturising and healing creams containing aloe vera and the natural antibiotic bee propolis.
Aloe vera gels: healing and conditioning gels for use on the face and body.
Aloe heat lotions: powerful and penetrating heat rubs—especially good for sports people.
Aloe moisturising lotions: the lotions have outstanding humectant and moisturising properties, and contain collagen and elastin to help keep the skin smooth, soft and elastic.

Key Points
The highest quality aloe vera lotions, gels and creams are formulated to incorporate the very latest advancements in fine skin care.

Soluble collagen, the major constituent of our connective tissue when we are young, is where skin ageing mainly occurs. This happens because as we grow older the soluble collagen becomes progressively more insoluble because of cross-linking within the collagenic fibrils.

This solubility provides the skin with good water absorption capacity due to the elasticity of the connective tissue. Older skin has less soluble collagen, and therefore less elasticity and less water absorption ability. This decrease is responsible for the physiological ageing process manifested by wrinkles and dry, aged-looking skin.

Elastin is the second most abundant constituent of the connective tissues. It has properties of elastic extension and contraction. As we grow older, elastin is also diminished in quality, leading to loss of flexibility of the skin and eventually wrinkling of the skin. Application of elastin in the moisturising lotion will enhance the flexibility of the epidermis because of its ability to bind moisture.

Aloe Activator: pure stabilised aloe vera gel with allantoin— an organic cell growth and renewal agent. It also contains methylparaben to preserve freshness and protect against microbial contamination. It is an excellent moisturising agent containing enzymes, amino acids and polysaccharides. It makes the ideal liquid partner to work synergistically with a Facial Contour Mask Powder to provide moisturisation, cleansing and controlled conditioning.

Washing, Cleansing and Conditioning

Aloe shampoos: mild, healing shampoos, can be used every day.

Aloe conditioners with jojoba: rich, healing conditioners, can be used every day.

Aloe soap: mild, no-tears formula liquid, very gentle cleanser.

Aloe deodorant: mild and effective, containing no aluminium salts.

Bath gelees: penetrating action with aloe vera that helps remove dead skin (with a loofah) and heals, soothes and stimulates the skin.

Aloe scrubs: exfoliating preparations made from an aloe vera base with natural jojoba beads as the abradant.

First Aid sprays: prepared from stabilised aloe vera gel with full-strength enzymes, amino acids, minerals and vitamins. These moisturising and healing products also contain allantoin, a skin protective ingredient occurring naturally in many plants, plus eleven natural herbs known for their soothing and healing properties.

Aftershave balms: with the healing properties of aloe vera.

Exfoliating cleaners: prepared from hypo-allergenic ingredients to provide a light, non-greasy, non-irritating lotion with balanced pH and moisture, for the effective removal of make-up, dirt, skin debris and grime.

Rehydrating toners: non-drying, non-alcohol formula containing natural aloe and witch hazel, special skin moisturisers, botanical extract for toning, and collagen and allantoin for structural and cell conditioning. It is a special stimulating formula, providing good secondary cleansing and toning to reduce pore size. Removes residual oils and dirt while invigorating the skin and leaving it clean, smoothed, balanced and stimulated.

Products for Mature Skin

Firming Foundation Lotion: specially formulated to be applied to the skin to firm, retexturise and tighten the pores while remoisturising the skin, re-establishing the lipid/moisture balance and providing a protective layer under make-up.

It contains a blend of aloe vera and other special moisturisers, humectants and conditioners plus collagen and elastin needed for maintaining good skin structure to restore a more youthful appearance. It also contains a protective factor that helps shield the skin from environmental hazards such as sunlight, wind and pollution, the accumulative effects of which can be the start of tired and wrinkled skin.

Night creams: designed for night use to restore the condition of the skin while the body is at rest restoring itself. They contain polysaccharides and other skin humectants to form a protective film against moisture loss.

They also contain special moisturisers such as aloe vera gel, sodium PCA, hyaluronic acid, glucose glutamate, sodium lactate and panthenol. Natural lipids for the important oil/water balance are provided by wheat germ glycerides, apricot kernel oil and jojoba oil. Soluble collagen and hydrolysed elastin are needed for maintaining good skin structure which helps combat the ageing look due to line and wrinkle formation. Special skin enhancers are derived from botanical and bee product extracts and allantoin.

R3 Factor Cream: helps promote smoother, younger-looking skin by reducing the appearance of lines and wrinkles on the skin's surface. R3 Factor contains free-radical scavengers (antioxidants) and moisture enhancers to provide protection from free-radical damage, plus the exfoliation of the top layer of the skin to produce a smoother, clearer texture. R3 Factor is designed to help counteract the signs of ageing. All the ingredients work together synergistically to help prevent and reduce facial lines, making the skin's appearance more youthful, softer and smoother.

Body Care

Aloe Lips: a healing salve.

Suntan Lotion: helps soothe, lubricate, moisturise and protect the skin.

Body Toning Kits: each kit contains an Aloe Body Toner for use with a cellophane wrap, an Aloe Body Conditioning Cream for non-wrap use and Aloe Bath Gelee to relax, smooth, and soothe the skin. A loofah is included for use in stimulating the skin during the bath.

Body toners: thick, emollient creams that contain aloe vera emulsifiers, moisturisers and humectants plus the circulatory and warming agents, cinnamon oil and capsicum.

Body conditioning creams: thick emollient emulsion with aloe vera, European herbal complexes, emulsifiers, humectants and conditioners. To be used as a massage cream between Body toner use, or as a spot rub or for entire hip and leg area.

Miscellaneous

Aloe Blossom Herbal Tea: a natural blend of international teas specially prepared to provide flavour and aroma. Designed to promote total relaxation and rest.

Multi-Purpose Detergent: a concentrated but mild laundry and general household cleaning product, designed to do the job of many conventional household products on the market. It must not be used in automatic dishwashers.

Aloe Pro-Set: a specially prepared hair spray whose main ingredients include stabilised aloe vera gel, purified water and hydrolysed vegetable protein. Purified water can protect and nourish hair, replenishing all the moisture lost due to sunlight or frequent blow drying. Stabilised aloe vera gel can increase the hair's elasticity and keep it soft and manageable. Hydrolysed vegetable protein replenishes lost nutrients.

Aloe toothgels: low abrasion toothgels combining the healing properties of aloe vera and bee propolis.

For Animal Use

Veterinary sprays: formulated from natural stabilised aloe vera gel, for its moisturising and anti-bacterial action. The aloe vera is complemented with allantoin, a natural wound healer that aids in the healing process.

Bibliography and References

Anderson, B.C. (1983). Aloe Vera Juice: A veterinary medicament? *The Compendium On Continuing Education for the Practising Veterinarian*, 5, S364–S368.

Bland, J. (1985). Effect of Orally Consumed Aloe Vera Juice on Gastrointestinal Function in Normal Humans, *Prevention*.

Buchman, D.D. (1983). *Herbal Medicine: The Natural Way to Get Well and Stay Well*, Rider.

Coats, B.C. and Holland, R.E. (1985). *Creatures in Our Care: The Veterinary Use of Aloe Vera*. Privately printed, Texas.

Coats, B.C. and Stephens, S. (1982). *Healing Winners*. Privately printed, Texas.

Coats, B.C. (1979). *The Silent Healer: A Modern Study of Aloe Vera*. Privately printed, Texas.

Courteney, H. (1996). *What's the Alternative?*, 2nd ed., Boxtree.

Danhof, I. *Remarkable Aloe*, video, PRO-MA Systems.

Editorial (1996). Aloe, aloe, *Country Living*.

El Zawahry, M., Hegazy, M.R. and Helal, M. (1973). Use of Aloe Vera in treating leg ulcers and dermatoses, *International Journal of Dermatology*, 12, 68073.

Gates, G. (1975). Aloe Vera—my favourite plant, *American Horticulturalist*, 54, 37.

Green, P. (1996). Aloe Vera Extracts in Equine Clinical Practice. *Veterinary Times*, 26, 9.

Gunther, R.T. (1934). *The Greek Herbal of Dioscorides*, Oxford University Press.

Heinerman, J. (1982). Aloe Vera, the Divine Healer, in *Aloe Vera, Jojoba and Yucca*, Keats Publishing.

Hennessee, O.M. and Cook, B.R. (1989). *Aloe Myth-Magic Medicine.*

Holford, P. (1992). *Optimum Nutrition,* ION Press.

Holford, P. (1996). *Living Food,* ION Press.

Morales, B.L. (n.d.). Aloe Vera, the miracle plant, reprinted from *Let's Live,* Health in Mind and Body, Los Angeles, California.

Northway, R.B. (1975). Experimental use of Aloe Vera extract in clinical practice. *Veterinary Medicine/Small Animal Clinician,* 70, 89.

Pietroni, P. (1995). *The Family Guide to Alternative Health Care,* Simon & Schuster.

Robson, M.C., Heggers, J.P. and Hagstrom, W.J. (1982). Myth, magic, witchcraft or fact? Aloe Vera revisited, *Journal of Burn Care and Rehabilitation,* 3, 157–163.

Sakai, R. (1989). Epidemiology Survey on Lung Cancer with Respect to Cigarette Smoking and Plant Diet, *Japanese Journal of Cancer Research.*

Skousen, M.B. *Aloe Vera Handbook,* Aloe Vera Research Institute, California.

Syed, T.A., Ashfaq, S., Holt, A.H., Ahmad, S.A., Ahmad, S.H. and Afzal, M. (1996). Management of psoriasis with *Aloe vera* extract in a hydrophilic cream: a placebo-controlled, double-blind study. *Tropical Medicine and International Health,* 1, 4, 505–509.

Taylor-Donald, L. (1980). Aloe Vera, 'The Wand of Heaven', *Bestways,* August.

Taylor-Donald, L. (1981). A Runner's Guide to Discovering the Secrets of the Aloe Vera Plant, *Runner's World,* December.

Trattler, R. (1987). *Better Health Through Natural Healing,* Thorsons.